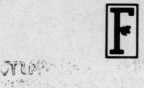

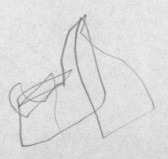

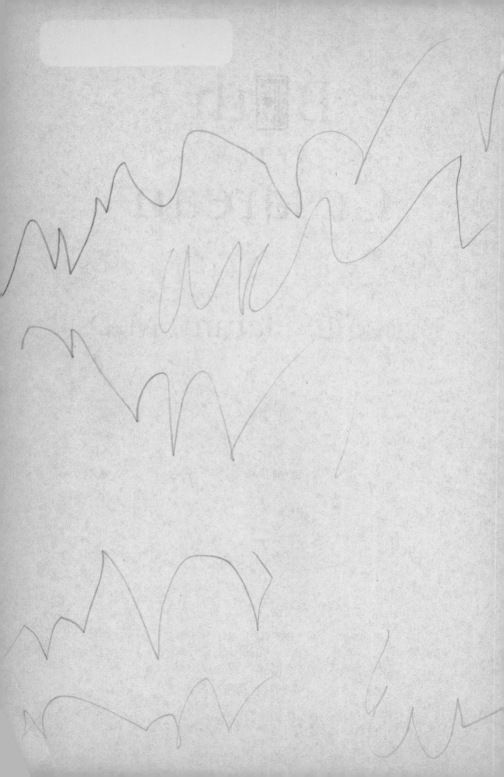

Birth
AFTER
Cesarean

THE MEDICAL FACTS

Bruce L. Flamm, M.D.

A FIRESIDE BOOK
Published by Simon & Schuster
New York   London   Toronto   Sydney
Tokyo   Singapore

FIRESIDE
Simon & Schuster Building
Rockefeller Center
1230 Avenue of the Americas
New York, New York 10020

First Fireside Edition 1992

FIRESIDE and colophon are registered trademarks
of Simon & Schuster Inc.

Designed by Barbara Cohen Aronica

Manufactured in the United States of America

10 9 8 7 6 5 4 3

Library of Congress Cataloging-in-Publication Data

Flamm, Bruce L.
    Birth after Cesarean / Bruce L. Flamm.
        p.   cm.
    Includes bibliographical references.
    1. Cesarean section—Complications and sequelae.   2. Natural
childbirth.   I. Title.
    RG761.F53   1990
    618.8'6—dc20   89-22900
                                                  CIP

ISBN 0-671-76187-0
ISBN 0-671-79218-0 (pbk)

The ideas, procedures, and suggestions contained in this book are not intended to replace the services of a trained health professional. All matters regarding your health require medical supervision. You should consult your physician before adopting the procedures in this book. Any applications of the treatments set forth in this book are at the reader's discretion.

The cases and examples cited in this book are based on actual situations and real people. Names and identifying details have been changed to protect privacy.

This book is dedicated to the one million American women who will have cesarean sections this year and to the millions of women who have already endured cesarean operations.

ACKNOWLEDGMENTS

The rapidly rising cesarean section rate is certainly not a popular topic among American obstetricians. The reasons for this are manifold, but suffice it to say that a doctor who speaks out on this controversial issue runs the risk of losing friends. So I would like to thank the wonderful people who have continued to support me in spite of my slightly heretical views!

Certain colleagues in particular stand out. Thanks to Ronald Kohorn, M.D., for setting a shining example of what it means to be a good doctor; Kenneth Bell, M.D., Medical Director, Kaiser-Permanente, Orange County, California, for never-ending support of my research endeavors; and Edward J. Quilligan, M.D., Editor of the American Journal of Obstetrics and Gynecology, for nurturing my early interest in vaginal birth after cesarean (VBAC).

I would also like to thank the many certified nurse-midwives who have, over the past eight years, constantly reminded me that pregnancy is *not* a disease but a normal physiological state. The VBAC mothers who graciously agreed to share their stories also deserve sincere gratitude.

Ms. Gail Winston, my editor at Prentice Hall Press, deserves special acknowledgment for having the foresight to immediately recognize the importance of VBAC.

Finally, I would like to thank the best midwife in the world, my wife, Janice Goings-Flamm, C.N.M., for putting up with me as I relentlessly cluttered the house with the thousand scraps of paper that would eventually become this book.

CONTENTS

FOREWORD

Ten years ago in our program at the University of California, a young resident (the author of this book) asked me to work with him on a paper concerning vaginal birth after cesarean section (VBAC). I was delighted to do so because I had been doing VBACs for twenty-five years and believed that they were safe. I didn't realize at the time that a force would be unleashed that would leave no stone unturned to get at the facts about birth after cesarean. The facts, which are being reinforced daily, are that VBAC is safe for both mother and child.

Simply stating that VBAC is safe for both mother and child should not be enough for an intelligent, questioning couple who achieve a pregnancy after having had a prior cesarean section. They should have questions—lots of them. Dr. Flamm, who has worked for the past seven years with couples who pose questions, has wisely chosen the question-and-answer format for his book. The result is an easy-to-read and valuable sourcebook which answers in an extremely factual and nonemotional way, almost all of the questions one could have about this procedure.

Being an obstetrician himself, Dr. Flamm has also given some very good advice on approaching your physician about VBACs. As he says, "Use a nonthreatening, nonjudgemental, intelligent approach." In other words, put yourself in your physician's chair. Remember, if someone demands something of you in a belligerent way, you resist; if a subject is discussed rationally you are more likely to go along with a request.

The only way the rapidly rising cesarean section rate will be reduced is to follow the recommendations given in this book. It should be required reading for every patient who is pregnant and has had a prior cesarean section, and for many of their obstetricians.

—Edward J. Quilligan, M.D.,
Editor, American Journal of
Obstetrics and Gynecology

PREFACE

In 1977, I learned a lesson that would change my life. I can still clearly recall the events of the day. I was a third-year medical student and was required to attend yet another noon lecture. I'd been at the hospital since about 5:00 A.M. and would have much rather headed for the cafeteria than the lecture hall. But the obstetric residents to whom I was assigned led the way and I did what medical students are supposed to do—I followed. The lecture hall quickly filled to capacity, mainly with men in long white jackets. These were the real doctors, either residents or staff physicians. A sprinkling of the audience, including myself, wore the short white coats of doctors-to-be.

The topic, which seemed rather esoteric to me at the time, was "vaginal birth after cesarean section." For the next hour I listened intently as a rather bold chief resident presented a list of arguments against routine repeat cesarean operations. He pointed out that the cesarean rate, which had been 5 percent in 1970, had tripled in less than ten years. He then reviewed medical reports dating back to the 1930s that seemed to indicate vaginal birth after cesarean section was both safe and likely to succeed. I was quite impressed. It seemed that this young doctor had clearly outlined a method by which many unnecessary operations could be safely avoided.

Much to my surprise the lecture was not well received. In fact, some of the comments that followed were downright hostile. I got the distinct feeling that the chief resident had trampled on hallowed ground. The lesson I learned that day was that there where things having to do with the practice of medicine that might not be found in medical textbooks. The fact that dozens of medical reports supported the safety and efficacy of vaginal birth after cesarean did not necessarily imply that it would be widely accepted. There were other factors involved that were not even mentioned in the books we medical students studied like bibles.

Over the next two years I witnessed a lot of cesarean sections, many that were routine repeat operations. But during all my years in medical school I never saw a woman give birth normally after a prior cesarean section. By the time I started my internship things were starting to change; at least at the large university hospitals, vaginal birth after cesarean section was becoming a fairly common event. My interest in cesarean section continued to grow. So did the cesarean rate. The year I attended the fateful lecture described above, just under half a million cesarean sections were performed in the United States. Ten years later the cesarean rate was approaching 25 percent and almost 1 million cesarean sections were being performed each year.

If present trends continue, there is a distinct possibility that some day the majority of American babies will be delivered by major surgery. I believe that this possibility is a frightening picture of technology gone awry. If we are to avoid this scenario steps must be taken to assure that each cesarean operation is a medically indicated operation. Through years of research I've come to the rather uncomfortable conclusion that the vast majority of routine repeat cesarean sections are simply not medically indicated. I believe that breaking the vicious cycle created by routine repeat cesarean sections is the only way we can get a handle on our runaway cesarean rate. It is my sincere hope that this book will help many women avoid unnecessary and potentially dangerous surgery.

INTRODUCTION

The Cesarean Controversy

Cesarean section is now the most common major operation performed in the United States. To say that our nation's increasing cesarean rate has become controversial would be a profound understatement. Dozens of local consumer groups and at least two national organizations have recently been formed to protest what has been termed a "cesarean crisis." What is the magnitude of this situation? In 1970, about 205,000 cesarean operations were performed in the United States, representing 5.5 percent of the total 3.7 million babies born. By 1987, 934,000 cesarean operations were performed in American hospitals. This fivefold increase took place despite the fact that the total number of births remained fairly constant at about 3.7 million per year. Thus, by 1987, 25 percent of all American babies were delivered by major surgery. Some experts believe that delivering one out of four babies by cesarean section is medically justified.

However, other authorities have presented strong arguments that at least half of these cesareans are not indicated, implying that one-half million unnecessary cesarean operations are being performed annually in the United States.

Critics of the rising cesarean rate have pointed out that one out of every three cesarean operations is performed solely because the mother has had a prior cesarean. These "routine repeat" cesareans account for almost a third of a million operations each year. After years of deliberation, the American College of Obstetricians and Gynecologists, the nation's largest organization of Ob-Gyn specialists, has recently recommended that with very few exceptions these "routine repeat" operations should no longer be performed. The organization recommends that these repeat operations be replaced by vaginal birth after cesarean (VBAC).

Although VBAC (pronounced "vee-back") has only recently become popular, the concept is certainly not a new one. For more than fifty years a few doctors have advocated allowing labor after a previous cesarean section. Their opinion was certainly not shared by the majority of obstetricians, at least not in the United States. Until the last few years only about one out of a hundred American women was allowed to attempt normal birth after cesarean section. A few medical reports have used the term vaginal delivery after cesarean (VDAC). It is true that a doctor performs the delivery if a baby is born by cesarean section. However, if a mother gives birth naturally, it is she, *not* the doctor, who gives birth. Hence, VBAC seems to be a more reasonable term. It has been estimated that if all eligible women attempted VBAC hundreds of thousands of cesarean operations could be safely avoided each year.

Not Just One Doctor's Opinion

From my personal experience with hundreds of "previous cesarean" mothers, I have come to the conclusion that for the majority of women normal birth after cesarean section is both safe and likely to succeed. (Although I will admit to having a personal bias in favor of attempting natural birth after cesarean, I've tried to not let it interfere with my objectivity.)

Cesarean section and normal birth after cesarean section may be controversial subjects, but some people go too far. For example, I've seen books that portray obstetricians as uncaring individuals who mercilessly seek any excuse to perform an operation. This type of vicious nonsense serves no purpose. However, it must be acknowledged that there are some obstetricians who, by distorting the risks of normal birth after cesarean section, continue to coerce women into unnecessary surgery. Neither these intractable doctors nor the irate childbirth activists who campaign against them can give a dispassionate view of birth after cesarean section. I'm convinced that the "truth" about the cesarean section controversy lies somewhere in between these two diametrically opposed points of view. This book offers a candid and thoroughly researched discussion of this topic; it does not represent one doctor's opinion.

I have personally reviewed the records of thousands of women who have experienced normal vaginal birth after a previous cesarean section. But the answers in this book are not derived from my own experience. No individual doctor has had enough experience with VBAC to draw reliable conclusions. The answers given in this book represent conclusions drawn from a thorough review of every medical publication written on the subject in the past fifty years. They represent the combined experience of literally hundreds of doctors from all over the world. Above all, the answers in this book represent a detailed analysis of the labors of more than ten thousand women who have given birth naturally in spite of their previous cesarean sections.

The reason this book strongly supports the concept of VBAC is because the bulk of recent medical research strongly supports VBAC. Unfortunately, many American obstetricians will still not allow normal birth after cesarean section.

I will attempt to explain why these doctors feel as they do. It is my sincere hope that this book will lead to a mutual understanding and cooperation between pregnant women and their doctors rather than serving as a source of hostility.

The Question-and-Answer Format

Today, perhaps more than ever before, most expectant mothers (and expectant fathers) lead hectic lives. In addition to running the household, most pregnant women in the United States work outside the home. At the end of a busy day you probably have much better things to do than drudging through a monotonous medical textbook. I started thinking about questions and answers as a learning tool about two years ago when I was teaching a VBAC class. This class started at 7:00 P.M. and I found that within the hour, half the people in the room weren't listening very attentively and the other half were gathering their things to leave.

I noticed, however, that every time I asked if anyone had questions, a strange thing would happen. Usually there was a tense pause until someone broke the ice by asking the first question. For example, a woman might ask why our hospital insists on fetal monitoring. Then hands would start to go up all over the place. Individuals who had been half asleep were suddenly sitting on the edge of their chair waving their hand! What had been a boring lecture was instantly transformed into an exciting two-way interaction. While I doubt that applying a question-and-answer format to this book will create quite the same excitement that it does in a room full of expectant parents, I do hope that this format will make things more interesting.

Another reason for this format is to allow you to quickly find the answer to a particular question without wading through pages of irrelevant information. For example, if your labor starts at 3:00 A.M. you're *not* going to want to start re-reading an entire book. You're going to want some quick answers to specific questions. That's exactly what you'll find in this book. Rather than rambling on about various subjects, each individual section is designed to thoroughly answer one specific question.

A third goal of the question-and-answer format is to allow you to skip from question to question as your time allows. Each question-answer pair is designed to be fairly independent so nothing will be lost if you choose to glance at a few pages on your lunch hour on Tuesday but don't get a chance to pick up the book again until Friday night.

Where did the questions come from? I spent almost a year thinking about things I might want to discuss with a cesarean couple if I had unlimited time. I wrote these things in a little notebook that I carried around in my pocket until it was almost too worn to read. Every few days I'd pull out the notebook and contemplate the list. Eventually I came up with almost twenty pages of questions. Every time I talked with a cesarean mother I'd check the list to see if anything was missing. Finally I asked several certified nurse-midwives and doctors to ask me questions about birth after cesarean section. When the time came that no one was asking me any questions that weren't already in my notebook, I decided that the list was complete.

Although I've tried to include every question that a reader might ask, I certainly wouldn't be surprised if some of you come up with new questions. If you do, I'd really like to hear from you. Please send any questions about VBAC to me at the following address: Bruce L. Flamm, M.D., c/o Fireside Books, Simon & Schuster, 1230 Avenue of the Americas, New York, NY 10020.

I can't promise to answer all the mail I receive but if you come up with a question I've missed, I'll include it along with a thoroughly researched answer in the next edition of this book. I'd also be interested in your comments about this book and about your experience with cesarean section and/or birth after cesarean section.

What This Book Can and Cannot Do

This book will answer almost any question you may have about normal birth after cesarean section. The risks and the benefits of VBAC will be thoroughly discussed so that you will be able to weigh all of your options. In addition to its function as a VBAC primer, this book will also explain many facets of the cesarean operation including its history, technique, and current indications. You will learn why the operation has become so common.

Perhaps the most important thing this book can offer is something that your physician cannot: unlimited time. Certainly, any doctor who has kept up with the current literature on birth after cesarean section might be able to provide reasonable answers to most of the questions in this book. But, let's face it, doctors are always pressed for time. In addition to the numerous questions that are likely to arise in any pregnancy, if a woman were to present her doctor with lists of questions about VBAC, it is unlikely that they would all be answered to her satisfaction. Unfortunately, even the most dedicated physician must place some limits on the amount of time he or she spends with each patient.

But it is certainly true that you deserve solid answers to your questions, especially when you are trying to decide whether or not to undergo major surgery. Since your questions also involve the health of your unborn child you certainly don't want to settle for someone's best guess or unsubstantiated opinion. You want *facts*. And that's exactly what you'll find in this book. There is also an appendix that offers complete references to dozens of medical reports from all over the world to validate the answers given here.

This book cannot tell you how to have your next baby. That decision can be made only by you, the parents, in conjunction with your doctor or midwife. This book will provide you with information that may help you with the decision-making process. However, it cannot force your doctor to go along with your wishes. It is quite possible that after reading this book and carefully weighing the alternatives you may decide not to undergo an automatic repeat cesarean operation. However, you may find that your doctor has no interest in any alternatives. Some possible solutions to this problem are offered here.

The Odds Are in Your Favor!

Many women would like to experience a normal birth after cesarean section but secretly doubt that they could succeed. They fear that they will get their hopes up only to end up with another cesarean operation. Many expectant parents have heard a little about VBAC but aren't at all sure about the odds. So let me begin by pointing out that the odds are in your favor! Many statistics will be discussed in detail later, but for now here are some encouraging results. In comprehensive medical studies of thousands of women attempting VBAC, about 70 percent to 80 percent were able to avoid repeat cesarean operations. In other words, approximately eight out of every ten women who attempt a vaginal birth after previous cesarean section will succeed.

Interestingly, even among women who had their initial cesarean because the baby wouldn't come out (pelvis supposedly too small, baby too big, cervix too stubborn, etc.), the majority will have a successful vaginal birth if they give it a try. Women with truly constricted pelvic bones are few and far between. Remember that the cesarean rate was 5 percent in 1970 and, unless an epidemic of deformed pelvic bones has mysteriously occurred, it is doubtful that women have suddenly lost the ability to give birth normally! The fact is that most women who attempt natural birth after cesarean section will succeed. This has been proven beyond a shadow of a doubt.

CHAPTER 1

Cesarean Section: Medical Facts

Is Cesarean Section a Common Operation?

Many people think that the most common major operation performed in the United States is the appendectomy or the tonsillectomy. However, cesarean section is the most frequently performed major operation in this country. Since 1983, it has never fallen out of first place.

In 1970, about 5 percent of the 3.7 million births in the United States were by cesarean section, which adds up to about 200,000 cesareans. That's a lot of operations but it's only the beginning of the story. By 1980, the cesarean rate had more than tripled (17 percent) and, in that single year, 619,000 American women had cesarean section operations. Some experts doubted that the trend could continue. They were wrong. In 1984, there were 813,000 cesareans performed in the United States. Amazingly, the rate continued to climb and, in 1986, 906,000 cesarean operations were recorded.

Initial estimates indicate that there were 934,000 cesarean operations performed in the United States during
1987, which means that 24.4 percent of all American babies were delivered by major surgery. To put it another
way, one out of every four women who walks into an
American hospital to have a baby now ends up on an
operating room table. Placing this statistic in context, it is
possible to compare these numbers to other commonly
performed operations. Since 1965, the National Center for
Health Statistics has published annual reports listing the
number of operations performed in American hospitals.[1]
The following table compares the number of major operations performed in 1965 to those performed in 1986:

	1965	1986	Change
Cesarean section	169,000	906,000	+436%
Hysterectomy	505,000	644,000	+ 27
Gall bladder removal	355,000	502,000	+ 41
Hernia repair	517,000	329,000	− 57
Tonsillectomy	1,215,000	281,000	− 332
Appendectomy	379,000	275,000	− 38
Mastectomy	266,000	132,000	− 102

By 1986, the number of cesarean operations was greater
than the combined total of all appendectomies, mastecto-
mies, and tonsillectomies!

Since it takes a great deal of time for government
agencies to compile national statistics we can only guess
how many cesareans are being done today. However, trends
over the past ten years make it almost certain that we will
soon exceed 1 million cesarean operations per year.

Is There a Cesarean Epidemic?

Although the term *epidemic* is generally used to describe a disease, other connotations exist. *Dorland's Medical Dictionary* defines epidemic as "attacking many people in any region at the same time; widely diffused and rapidly spreading." In addition to its usual disease-related meaning, *Webster's Dictionary* also defines epidemic as "the rapid, widespread occurrence of a fad, fashion, etc." Since the incidence of cesarean operations has been increasing rapidly over widespread areas, it would seem fair to conclude that we are in the midst of a cesarean epidemic.

Figures 1 and 2 show the increase of cesarean sections in the United States over the past fifteen to twenty years. You don't need a degree in mathematics to see that something amazing happened around 1970! For generations the cesarean section rate in the United States had remained below 5 percent. Then between 1970 and 1978, in a time span of only eight years, the cesarean section rate tripled. The rate, which had been about 5 percent in 1970, increased 300 percent to more than 15 percent in 1978.

Although the national cesarean section rate is now almost 25 percent, some hospitals have higher cesarean rates than others. The *Los Angeles Times* recently reported that twenty-three Southern California hospitals had cesarean section rates greater than 33 percent.[2] At these hospitals at least one out of every three infants is surgically removed!

In the past ten years approximately 6 million American women have undergone the cesarean operation. This number is greater than the entire combined female populations of the states of Alaska and Maine! More women have had cesarean operations in the past ten years than in the prior thirty years combined even though the total number of births has recently declined. Overall, approximately 15 million living American women have undergone the cesarean operation. This number is now increasing by almost 1 million per year.

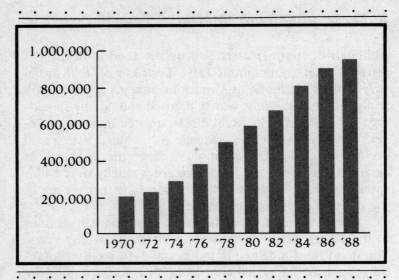

Figure 1. Biannual totals of cesarean sections in the United States since 1970.

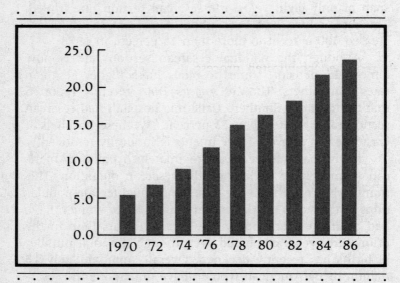

Figure 2. Biannual percentage of cesarean sections per total births in the United States since 1970.

Why Doesn't Somebody Do Something?

When an epidemic disease breaks out in this country several government agencies swing into action. Whether the offender is contaminated cheese or venereal disease, divisions of the Public Health Department or the Centers for Disease Control in Atlanta are on the move the instant an epidemic is even suspected. Although the rapid increase in cesareans may be considered an epidemic, it is an epidemic of operations, not an epidemic of disease. Thus, it creates several rather unusual situations. First, whose job is it to investigate a runaway operation: A state board of medical quality assurance? The Centers for Disease Control? A senate subcommittee? A federal agency?

Second, does the situation need investigation at all? One out of every four American babies is now delivered by the cesarean operation, but is that a problem? Many doctors don't seem to think so. Apparently the U.S. government did feel that the situation warranted investigation. In 1979, just after the cesarean rate had tripled, the National Institutes of Health (NIH) selected a nineteen-member Task Force on Cesarean Childbirth. In fall 1979, the task force began the complicated process of reviewing the volatile cesarean situation. One year later, in September 1980, a major conference was held at the NIH headquarters in Bethesda, Maryland. The task force spent the next year evaluating the recommendations of health-care professionals and representatives from the lay public. In October 1981, the results of the task force investigation were published in a 537-page report entitled "Cesarean Childbirth."[3]

Although many of the conclusions made in the report are beyond the scope of this book, it is worth noting that some of their major recommendations had to do with VBAC. The report revealed that "In 1978, 98.8 percent of all pregnant women with a previous cesarean were delivered surgically." Only about 1 percent of American women with prior cesarean sections were being allowed to give birth naturally. After twenty-seven pages of statistics and discussion about VBAC, the report concluded that "Based on maternal and neonatal mortality rates, the practice of routine repeat cesarean birth is open to question. Repeat cesarean carries two times the risk for maternal mortality (mother's death) of vaginal delivery." Finally, the government report encouraged doctors to allow their patients with prior cesareans to attempt normal vaginal birth.

With elective repeat cesarean section still being so common today one might wonder if the government report was kept secret. To the contrary, the report generated quite a bit of commotion. One way to access how important an issue is, or at least how controversial it is, would be to see how much press coverage it generates. The Rand Corporation conducted a massive study of newspapers and magazines across the country to see what was being printed about medical issues. The final results of the detailed computer search, which ended in 1982, were published in the *Journal of the American Medical Association*.[4] The study showed that of all the medical topics investigated by the U.S. government, none generated more interest than cesarean section. Even popular topics like breast cancer and heart bypass surgery received less press coverage. In fact, eighty-nine articles on cesarean section were found between 1980 and 1984, and sixty-six of these discussed the NIH Task Force report. What was the result of all this publicity? Essentially nothing.

Almost ten years have passed since this major NIH study strongly recommended that doctors utilize VBAC as one method of controlling America's skyrocketing cesarean section rate. However, the NIH apparently has no power to enforce its recommendations. Today, in spite of governmental recommendations to the contrary, nine out of ten cesarean mothers will undergo elective repeat cesarean operation if they choose to have more children.

Is a Cesarean Section a Major Operation?

Absolutely. Doctors often divide operations into two types: major and minor. Major operations include procedures done on internal organs such as the heart, brain, bowel, or female reproductive organs. Minor operations include procedures such as biopsies (taking samples of tissue), simple cosmetic procedures, and dilation and curettage (D and C). Major operations generally imply major risk; minor operations imply lesser risk.

Cesarean section has become so commonplace that some people seem to equate the magnitude of the operation with getting one's ears pierced! I recently had one patient with no prior cesarean section ask if she could just have a "C" because her first labor had been rather difficult. Another pregnant patient recently told me that she wanted her tubes tied after her baby was born. She requested that I "just do a section" and tie her tubes at the same time.

If there is any doubt in your mind, let's clear the air right now. Cesarean section is a major operation. It involves cutting through all layers of the abdominal wall and entering the body cavity that contains vital internal organs such as the stomach and intestines. It is remarkable that this operation has become so commonplace that the same woman who would cringe at the thought of an appendectomy might cheerfully accept a recommendation for a (perhaps unnecessary) repeat cesarean operation.

In reality, the layers of tissue cut through to reach an internal organ, be it the womb or the appendix, are just about identical. However, there is one major difference. Since your appendix is only about the size of your little finger, the opening required to remove it is usually only about two inches long. In contrast, the cesarean incision must be large enough to accommodate a typical twenty-inch-long infant weighing seven or eight pounds!

How Is the Operation Performed?

Dorland's Medical Dictionary defines cesarean section as "incision through the abdominal and uterine walls for delivery of a fetus." First, anesthesia is administered. The preferred form of anesthesia is *regional*, either spinal or epidural so the medications do not enter the mother's bloodstream and hence don't affect the baby. At times, either because time is of the essence or because no one is available to administer regional anesthesia, general anesthesia is used, which means that the mother is put totally to sleep. In addition to subjecting the baby to at least some dose of powerful hypnotic drugs, this method also destroys any chance of early bonding since the mother does not usually awaken until long after the infant has been delivered.

Next the mother's abdomen is cleansed and the skin incision is made. Today, by far the most common type of skin incision is a transverse cut made along the pubic hairline. Some doctors still prefer to make a vertical skin incision extending from the belly button to the pubic bone. However, since this up-and-down incision leaves a disfiguring scar, and since it offers no clear-cut advantages over the more cosmetic "bikini" incision, there is little justification for its continued use.

The next step is to cut through the fatty layer beneath the skin. Then the two layers of leatherlike fascia are cut open and the muscles that guard the abdomen are separated. Finally, the thin covering of the internal organs (peritoneum) is cut open. At this point the uterus (womb) and other internal organs such as the bowel and bladder come into view.

Next the bladder is carefully cut away and a transverse incision is made in the lower part of the uterus. The uterine incision is widened and the infant is delivered through the incision by pushing down on the mother's upper abdomen.

After delivering the placenta (afterbirth), the second

half of the operation begins. This step involves the repair of all of the layers mentioned above. First, the hole in the uterus is repaired with two layers of sutures each consisting of about ten stitches. Next, the bladder is sewn back into place with a fine row of stitches. Then the peritoneum is closed and the two layers of fascia are sewn back together. Finally, the skin is put back together either with sutures or with metal staples.

Patients often ask how many stitches are required during a cesarean section. Although the number certainly varies from operation to operation, a rough estimate would be about fifty or sixty.

What Is a Low Transverse Cesarean Section?

This operation, sometimes called a low segment cesarean, is the operation as described above. Today the vast majority of cesareans are of this type; the chances are at least nine out of ten that you had this type of surgery. In this operation, the very lowest portion of the womb is opened from side to side. VBAC is safe after this type of cesarean.

What Is a Classical Cesarean Section?

This surgery will be discussed more thoroughly in the section on the history of the operation, but briefly a classical cesarean involves an incision in the uterus (womb) that extends vertically from top to bottom. Another unusual type of cesarean is called the low vertical in which the uterine incision is also up and down rather than transverse.

With the low vertical type of uterine incision, attempting a subsequent vaginal birth may be dangerous, although some recent reports disagree. With a classical uterine incision, attempting vaginal birth is definitely dangerous. However, there are two important points to remember.

First, both the classical and the low vertical incisions are now rare. The classical cesarean section procedure began to diminish in use in the 1920s and by 1951 a medical report concluded that "Except for a small group of patients who present mechanical difficulty such as cervical myomas, we believe that classic cesarean section is an outmoded, obsolete, and dangerous operation."[5] Today, the vast majority of all cesareans are of the common low transverse type. Unless your first cesarean was done because of a transverse lie (baby coming down sideways) or unless your baby was very premature (on the order of two pounds) it is highly unlikely that you had anything but the common low transverse cesarean.

Second, these terms apply only to the incision on the uterus (womb), not to the skin incision. Therefore, even if you have an up-and-down skin incision, it is most likely that you have a low transverse (safe) uterine incision. Some older doctors who trained before the "bikini age" still prefer to make up-and-down skin incisions. Although the scar that results is less cosmetic, it does not make VBAC dangerous. Remember, a vertical skin scar does not imply that you had a classical cesarean section. It is the scar on the uterus, not the scar on the skin, that is important when considering vaginal birth after cesarean section.

How Do I Find Out Which Type of Cesarean I Had?

Most hospitals will be happy to give you information contained in the hospital chart compiled when you had your cesarean section. In fact, I've never seen a hospital refuse to do so. However, for legal reasons, the hospital must be careful in sending out information from your chart. They must be certain that it is indeed you and not some other prying individual who is trying to gain access to your records. For this reason, many hospitals are reluctant to give out information over the phone.

Most hospitals require that you obtain a form for release of information from your current doctor. Note that it is not necessary to request the entire chart. Your chart may be a hundred pages long, and you may be charged unnecessary copying fees if you don't specify exactly what you need. You should simply request the operative report. Be sure to give your full name and the date of the cesarean operation. Of course, the date is easy to remember since it is your baby's birthday.

When this page arrives it will generally specify that you had a low transverse or low segment cesarean, because in recent years the classical type of cesarean section has become almost obsolete. In the rare event that the report states you had a classical or low vertical uterine incision, most doctors would recommend that you do not attempt a vaginal birth.

If for some reason the hospital medical records department does not quickly provide the necessary information by mail, your doctor may be able to solve the problem with a simple phone call. As explained above, most hospitals prefer not to give out information over the phone. However, if your due date is approaching and the answer has not come back in the mail, or if you go into premature labor, there may be no time to wait. I have found that confirmation of previous cesarean section scar type is becoming such a common request that most medical record personnel will quickly respond to a personal phone call from a physician. On several occasions I've had patients whose first cesarean section was performed in another country. I've called and talked (at times with the help of a translator) with medical record personnel all over the world and I've never encountered a hospital that would not read me the relevant information over the phone.

Don't put off this matter until your ninth month! Some women prefer to obtain the operative report even before they get pregnant again.

What Is a Primary Cesarean Section?

A woman's operative report will most often begin with the phrase "primary low transverse cesarean section." The word *primary* has caused some people a great deal of concern.

Primary can signify "critical"; however, "primary cesarean section" simply means the *first* cesarean section. The word implies nothing about how or why the operation was done or about how many children you've had. Even if you've had three prior natural births, the first cesarean section is still called a primary cesarean section.

Any cesarean that is not a primary one is called a repeat cesarean. At many hospitals it is still assumed that any woman who gets pregnant after having a primary cesarean section will automatically have a repeat cesarean.

What Is an Elective Repeat Cesarean Section?

An elective repeat cesarean section is a repeat cesarean operation that has no specific indication for being performed. In contrast, a primary cesarean section must always have an indication. It would be highly unusual for a doctor to perform a primary cesarean section without clearly stating why the procedure was being done. The reason for doing a first cesarean section is generally stated at the very top of the operative report. For example, if you were to read the operative report from your primary cesarean section you would probably find the words "primary cesarean section for failure to progress in labor" or "primary cesarean section for breech." No doctor would report an elective primary cesarean section. In contrast, elective (unindicated) repeat cesarean section has been quite acceptable.

The term *elective*, defined as "that which is chosen but not required," clearly implies a choice. However, at least until recently, it was not the pregnant woman who was doing the choosing! In the past, the vast majority of women were not even informed of the option of vaginal birth after cesarean section. So to call the repeat operation "elective" or "optional" seems ludicrous. In any case, this terminology has persisted for decades.

Today many doctors feel that elective repeat cesarean sections should be abandoned. They feel that every cesarean operation, repeat as well as primary, should be required to have a specific indication. For example, a legitimate repeat operation might be reported as "repeat cesarean section done because the initial cesarean was of the classical type." Another example of an indicated or nonelective repeat cesarean section would be "repeat cesarean performed on polio victim because she is physically unable to give birth vaginally." The American College of Obstetrics and Gynecology has recently stated that "The concept of routine repeat cesarean section should be replaced by a *specific indication* for a subsequent abdominal delivery."[6]

Amazingly, the single most common reason for cesarean section in the United States today is "elective" repeat. Almost 300,000 elective repeat cesarean operations are performed every year in this country.

Is There Any Difference Between a Primary and a Repeat Cesarean Section?

A primary (first) cesarean section is generally a rather easy operation to perform. By easy I don't mean to imply risk-free. As was discussed previously, any cesarean section is a major operation and any major operation can result in major complications. But in terms of the technical difficulty, a primary cesarean section is usually easier to perform than a repeat cesarean, because scar tissue formation, or adhesions, are not a complication. In the hospital where I was trained there was a rule regarding cesarean sections: Interns could not even assist on repeat operations.

During a primary cesarean section, the tissue layers generally separate smoothly. In contrast, during a repeat operation the tissues are often fused together with old scar tissue. This scar tissue is often so thick and difficult to cut through that doctors call it "cement." The internal scar tissue rarely causes any health problems but it can make repeat operations a real challenge. Because of the scar tissue, the risk of injury to the bowel or bladder is definitely higher in repeat cesarean operations.

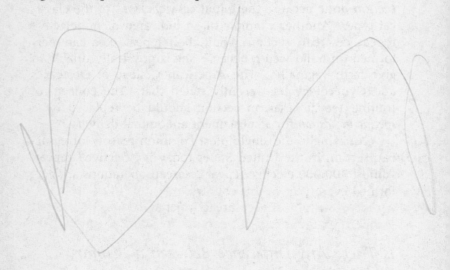

CHAPTER 2

A Brief History of the Cesarean Operation

When Was the First Cesarean Section Performed?

Crude forms of the cesarean operation have been performed for hundreds of years in an effort to save infants from dead mothers. The first cesarean performed on a living woman is reported to have occurred in 1500 when Jocob Nufer, a Swiss hog gelder, operated on his wife during an obstructed labor.[1] Mrs. Nufer apparently lived. Prior to the mid-1800s, there are only a few poorly documented reports of cesarean operations performed on living women, because most often the woman would die as a result of the surgery. For example, in England in 1865, nine out of ten mothers would die from complications of cesarean. At about the same time in France, not a single woman had survived the cesarean operation.

The cesarean operation has become so commonplace today that it's astounding to realize that just one hundred years ago the operation was almost uniformly fatal! Prior to this century, most mothers died after cesarean section from either hemorrhage or overwhelming infection. Two major breakthroughs in medicine—blood transfusion and powerful antibiotics—have vastly decreased these risks. However, even with all our modern technology, a mother is still more likely to die from complications of a cesarean section than from complications of a vaginal birth. Since cesarean section is now the method of delivery for one out of every four American babies, it is interesting to reflect that the human race survived for countless generations without the operation.

When Was the First Cesarean Section Performed in the United States?

Doctor Jesse Bennett supposedly performed the cesarean operation on his wife in 1794; however, some experts feel that this story is false. Hence, the first documented cesarean in the United States was done by Doctor John Richmond of Newton, Ohio, in April 1827.[2]

In 1849, a major obstetrics textbook was published by Dr. Charles Meigs, one of the fathers of American obstetrics and gynecology.[3] In his book, Dr. Meigs stressed that the cesarean operation was so incredibly dangerous that it should almost never be performed. He felt that the one and only indication for this operation was the rare case in which the mother would die without it. As explained in the following quotation, Dr. Meigs felt that even if the baby's life was in danger, the operation was far too dangerous to attempt unless the mother's life was also in danger:

> The cesarean operation, in its spirit and intention, should be devoted absolutely to the conservation of the mother alone. In saying so, I am not insensible of the great satisfaction to be enjoyed by that surgeon

who, under the distressing duress which should alone compel him to subject a living woman to the cesarean section, is rewarded with the happiness of rescuing both the child and its parent from the jaws of an otherwise inevitable grave. I hold that no man has a right to subject a living, breathing, human creature to so great a hazard as that attending the cesarean section, from views relating to any other interests than those of his patient.

Prior to 1850, doctors didn't realize the importance of sewing up the uterus after the baby was removed. Very few women survived. Even after the technique of closing the womb was discovered the operation remained treacherous. A report of seventeen cesareans done with this new method in the United States between 1852 and 1880 revealed that nine of the seventeen mothers died.

The classical technique began to be replaced by a low vertical method in the early 1920s. The low transverse cesarean in common use today was suggested by Dr. Kerr in 1926.[4] By 1933, the chance of a mother dying from the operation was reduced to about one in ten. Today, thanks to powerful antibiotics and other scientific innovations, the risk of a mother dying as a result of cesarean operation is extremely low. However, as we will see later, the risk remains higher than with normal vaginal delivery.

How Did the Operation Get Its Name?

Surprisingly, no one knows where the name for this operation came from! Williams' textbook of obstetrics lists three theories for possible origins of the name.[5]

The most commonly held belief is that Julius Caesar was born by this method and hence *cesarean* came from his name. However, this theory is almost certainly not true. Caesar was born around 100 B.C. and historians note that his mother not only survived the birth but lived for quite some time afterward. But since no woman was reported to have survived the operation until about 1100—centuries after Caesar's birth—it is almost impossible that he could have been delivered surgically. Note, however, that the British still use the spelling *caesarean.*

Another theory has to do with a Roman law that supposedly existed hundreds of years before Julius Caesar's time. If a pregnant woman died, this law called the *Lex Caesarea* mandated that her abdomen be opened and the infant removed. In those days the operation was invariably fatal so it was only performed on women who were already dead.

A final explanation, and the most probable, is that the term cesarean section was derived hundreds of years after Caesar's death from the two Latin words *caedere* and *seco.* Since both of these words mean "to cut" it seems that *cesarean section* is redundant. It literally means "cut-cut."

Why Was the Cesarean Operation Originally Performed?

Originally the operation was used only to removed a fetus from a dead mother. At times this surgery was done soon after the mother's death in an attempt to save the baby. Later the operation was performed on living women but only when it was absolutely impossible for the baby to be born vaginally. It should be stressed that the cesarean operation was developed as a radical intervention to assist the *rare* woman who was physically incapable of giving birth naturally. A report in 1879 revealed that the operation had been performed on sixteen dwarfs because of pelvic deformity and eleven of the sixteen women died from the surgery.[6]

As the operation became safer the restrictions on its use were relaxed. Originally used only as a last resort, cesarean section has become a "cure" for almost any problem that develops during labor. A recent medical article listed twenty-six indications for why a cesarean section might be performed.[7]

Once a Cesarean, Always a Cesarean?

Every obstetrician is familiar with the old rule "once a cesarean, always a cesarean." Most doctors know that this rule is no longer true. In fact, in 1984 the president of the American College of Obstetrics and Gynecology, Dr. Luella Klein, stated that it was an "outmoded dictum."[8] Unfortunately, some obstetricians continue to enforce the obsolete rule.

But where did the rule come from? Was the doctor who coined the phrase just trying to increase the number of cesareans? No. In fact, just the opposite is true! In July 1916, Dr. Edwin B. Cragin published an article in the *New York Medical Journal*.[9] The article was actually an attack on doctors who resorted to radical and unnecessary obstetric surgery.

To anyone who reads the essay, it is clear that Dr. Cragin used the phrase "Once a cesarean, always a cesarean" to stress that one of the main dangers of the operation was that it might have to be repeated. In those days, if the first cesarean didn't kill the mother a repeat operation very well could have! Hence, he used the phrase not as an argument against VBAC but to support his contention that no cesarean operation should be performed unless it is absolutely necessary. In fact, in the same paper he reported that one of his own patients had three VBACs without any difficulty! Unfortunately, some doctors chose to pull the now-famous six words out of context and ignore what Dr. Cragin actually said. In any case, neither VBAC nor repeat cesarean section was a major issue in 1916 since less than 1 percent of women had cesareans. (The rate is twenty-five times higher today!)

Another essential point to remember is that in 1916 almost all cesareans were of the classical type. As explained elsewhere in this book, the classical cesarean weakens the uterus to such an extent that subsequent natural birth would be risky. However, today, the classical cesarean is rarely performed.

CHAPTER 3

The Cesarean
Operation Today

Why Are So Many Cesarean Sections Performed Today?

If you asked five different doctors this question, you would probably get five different answers. I don't mean to imply any lack of candor but rather that there actually are many different reasons for the rising rate. For example, ten years ago most breech babies were delivered vaginally. Today, the majority of breech babies are delivered by cesarean section. Many doctors fear that a breech baby's head will be trapped after the legs and torso have been delivered. Although uncommon, this situation is dangerous to the baby. Hence, many doctors insist on delivering all breech babies by cesarean section. But since only about 3 or 4 percent of babies are upside-down at term, breech babies can only explain a very small part of our nation's skyrocketing cesarean rate.

Another reason for the rising rate has been fetal distress. Fetal monitors have only been around for about twenty years. These monitors aren't perfect, and the interpretation of fetal monitoring is a very inexact science. Sometimes an emergency cesarean section is performed because a fetal monitor seems to indicate fetal distress and yet the baby turns out to be perfectly healthy with no sign of distress. Some doctors would argue that the explanation of such cases is that the monitor caught things just in time. Others might argue that the monitor was in error! In any case, fetal distress only accounts for a small percentage of all cesarean sections and thus, like breech, is only responsible for a very small portion of the rising cesarean section rate.

Another recent indication for performing the cesarean operation is genital herpes. In adults, herpes usually causes a recurrent skin infection that is often painful but almost never dangerous. In contrast, when it occurs in a newborn, the virus can cause serious damage. The important thing to remember is that herpes infection in the newborn is rare even among women with genital herpes. Unfortunately, we cannot yet reliably predict which herpes-infected mothers will pass the virus to their infants. Hence, some misguided doctors have made it a rule to perform cesarean sections on all women with genital herpes.

One of the largest contributors to the rising cesarean section rate is dystocia, or abnormal labor. Dystocia encompasses many other medical terms such as cephalopelvic disproportion (CPD) and failure to progress in labor (FTP). In any case, these terms imply that for one reason or another the labor is not progressing at a normal rate. However, just what constitutes a "normal" rate of progress in labor is open to interpretation. Suffice it to say that in recent years it has become quite common to see a cesarean section performed simply because the cervix has not dilated much in an hour or two.

All of the above reasons for the rising cesarean section rate are discussed in obstetrics textbooks. However, fear of a lawsuit—perhaps the most important reason—is almost never discussed. When a doctor performs a cesarean section for fetal distress, herpes, or dystocia, he or she may be quite aware that the baby would be in almost no jeopardy from a natural birth. However, the doctor also knows that if anything goes wrong, and a cesarean section was not performed, an explanation will be necessary. A common saying among obstetricians is, "The only cesarean I've ever been sued for is the one I didn't do." It is unfortunate but true that until something can be done about misguided lawsuits, the cesarean section rate is not likely to fall.

Is the Cesarean Rate Still Increasing?

Yes. The National Institutes of Health (NIH) Task Force report on cesarean section covered 1970 to 1978. A staggering increase in the cesarean rate from 5.5 percent in 1970 to 15 percent in 1978 was reported.[1] This threefold increase might not seem like much until you remember that about 3.5 million babies are born in this country every year, which translates to an additional 350,000 women who will have the operation!

The NIH Task Force reported that 195,000 cesarean operations were performed in 1970. By 1978, the number had increased to 510,000 operations! Can't the increase be at least partially explained by the fact that many more babies were born in 1978 than in 1970? No. In fact, the total number of births had actually fallen by 1978.

But what's happened since 1978? In 1979, 601,000 cesareans were performed. By 1981, the number had increased to 704,000. In 1983, 809,000 cesarean operations were performed in the United States. The most recent national data are still being tabulated so it's hard to say exactly how many cesarean operations are being done today. However, some interesting data are available. In July 1985, the *Register*, a large California newspaper, investigated the hospital maternity services in Orange County, which is Los Angeles County's southern neighbor.[2] Data on the 1984 cesarean section rates were obtained from fifteen hospitals. The rates varied 18 percent to 30 percent.

The 30 percent figure wasn't the result of a knife-happy doctor at an isolated hospital. In reality, five of the fifteen hospitals had cesarean rates of more than 28 percent. For the entire group of fifteen hospitals there were 26,189 deliveries in 1984. Overall, 6,184, or 24 percent, of these babies were delivered by cesarean sections.

An extensive report on the rising cesarean section rate in the United States was recently released by the Public Citizen Health Research Group in Washington, D.C. This document provides statistics from forty-one states.[3] The report lists more than one hundred hospitals with cesarean rates of 35 percent or greater. At one hospital in Florida, 53 percent of all babies were delivered by cesarean! The Health Research Group report concludes that half of the 934,000 cesarean sections done in the United States in 1987 were unnecessary. The report also concludes that if women with a previous cesarean section had been encouraged to deliver vaginally in subsequent pregnancies, at least 237,000 cesarean sections performed in 1987 could have been avoided.

Why the Sudden Interest in Vaginal Birth after Cesarean (VBAC)?

For many years having a cesarean section meant that any future babies would require additional surgery. Why is this situation changing? There are at least five reasons for the recent interest in VBAC.

First, the American cesarean section rate is climbing at a staggering rate. Prior to the 1970s, it was unusual for a labor to end with a cesarean section. In fact, only three or four women out of a hundred (3 percent to 4 percent) had the cesarean operation. Hence, the total number of women who might be candidates for VBAC was relatively small. But in the 1970s, the cesarean section rate suddenly tripled. With 15 percent of all babies being delivered by the cesarean operation, the number of women with cesarean scars began to increase rapidly. The national cesarean section rate has now reached about 25 percent, meaning that almost a million cesarean sections are performed in the United States each year. Today, there are literally millions of women walking around with cesarean section scars. Many of these women will choose to have more children and would prefer to avoid additional surgery.

A second reason for the sudden interest in VBAC is the growing number of medical studies that support the safety of normal birth after cesarean section. More than fifty such studies have been published in the past thirty years. Many of these studies will be discussed later in this book.

Third, a change in the way the cesarean operation is performed has made VBAC safer, and thus it is more common. Years ago the operation was done through an up-and-down incision and the uterus (womb) was more likely to rupture. But this classical type of cesarean section has become almost obsolete.

Fourth, with the cost of health care now soaring, insurance companies may refuse to pay for operations that are not necessary. It is also true that many young couples do not have adequate health insurance coverage. For such families, an extra two or three thousand dollars added to the hospital bill may be a very heavy financial burden.

A final reason for the current interest in VBACs is the rise in consumerism. In recent years, individuals have been increasingly inclined to investigate all alternatives in their health care and to insist on having a more active role in the decision-making process.

How Many Cesarean Sections Can I Have?

As was previously explained, repeat cesarean sections can be more dangerous than primary (first) cesarean sections.

Because of the buildup of adhesions (internal scar tissue), repeat operations can become successively more difficult. Some obstetricians also believe that multiple cesarean sections weaken the uterus. Thirty years ago the concern about multiple repeat cesarean sections was so great that it was common practice to sterilize a woman after two or three cesarean sections.[4]

A medical report from England included discussion of a woman who died at the time of her fourth elective repeat cesarean section.[5] The report cautioned that "There are considerable risks attached to multiple cesarean sections and it is recommended that the operation be undertaken by consultant staff."

As will be discussed later, multiple repeat cesarean sections also predispose a woman to a dangerous condition called placenta previa accreta. In this condition, because the placenta (afterbirth) cannot be separated from the uterus, a hysterectomy is generally required.

Many doctors feel that because of these risks women should limit their number of cesarean sections. This can create a real conflict for a couple who desires a large family. One way to avoid this potential conflict is to remember that there does not seem to be any increased risk involved with having several normal births after a cesarean section. While there is some risk associated with repetitive cesarean operations, there does not appear to be any additional risk involved with repetitive VBACs.

CHAPTER 4

Risks of Vaginal Birth after Cesarean (VBAC)

If I Choose VBAC, What Are the Risks to My Baby?

When contemplating a VBAC many women have one overriding concern: Will attempting a vaginal birth put the baby in danger? It is important to remember that no doctor has had enough experience with VBAC to answer this question. For example, Dr. Jones in New York City may have observed the labors of twenty-seven women with previous cesareans during his career. If all of those babies were delivered safely, would that prove that VBAC was totally safe? Of course not. Only by reviewing the data from hundreds of doctors in hospitals all over the world can a statistically valid answer be reached.

But how many VBAC results need to be considered? One hundred? Five hundred? A thousand? No one knows for sure, but the more data collected, the more likely it is that the true risks involved will be determined. Insurance companies have used this method for years. If they want to know what the chances of death are for a sixty-four-year-old truck driver who smokes two packs of cigarettes a day, they study hundreds or thousands of these men rather than just a few.

Using a medical library computer to review the medical literature, I was able to come up with a list of forty-three reports in the medical journals during the thirty-five-year period from 1950 to 1985. These papers reported on a total of 11,027 women who had attempted VBAC: 8,693, or 78.8 percent, of these women had successful vaginal births in spite of their previous cesarean operations.

As far as risks to the baby, there were two fetal deaths per ten thousand births due to low transverse uterine rupture. Thus, the risk of a baby dying because of uterine rupture appears to be less than one in one thousand. To put these numbers in perspective, remember that in the United States the perinatal mortality rate is around 1.1 percent.* In other words, if a woman decides to have a natural birth after a previous cesarean section, she is essentially at no higher risk of losing her baby than any other woman.

A few other fetal losses occurred in the 11,027 VBAC attempts discussed above, but these were due to rupture of a prior classical uterine incision. These mothers certainly would not have been allowed a trial of labor today. One woman had a prior low vertical uterine incision. Another woman was treated with vaginal prostaglandin pessaries, a strong labor stimulant that would not be used today in a woman with a previous cesarean section. Finally, most of the women in these studies had their VBACs prior to the era of fetal monitoring.

Three recent studies are far larger than previous reports. In a University of Southern California study, reporting on more than a thousand trials of labor, not a single

---

*Most of these babies die due to premature labor or birth defects. This figure sounds scary, but remember that 99 percent of all pregnancies result in normal, healthy babies.

baby was lost due to rupture of a low transverse incision.[1] In a study that I conducted involving ten California hospitals there were 1,776 trials of labor without a single fetal loss due to uterine rupture.[2] Finally, doctors from Dublin, Ireland, recently reported on 1,781 trials of labor over a six-year period.[3] There was one fetal death apparently due to scar rupture. Thus, of the three recent major studies, only one baby was lost out of more than five thousand trials of labor. To put this number in perspective, we must remember that the American perinatal mortality rate is about ten per one-thousand births. Thus, according to recent studies, the risk of infant mortality as a result of a ruptured uterus is fifty times less than the risk of dying from other causes.

If I Choose VBAC, What Are the Risks to Me?

Perhaps the most common concerns about VBAC have to do with its safety. Women (and their husbands) contemplating birth after cesarean want to know what risks are involved. Unfortunately the information often given to potential VBAC candidates has not been thorough or accurate.

I recently met a woman who claimed her doctor said that VBAC might kill her. Even if she survived her baby would probably die and she would probably end up with a hysterectomy! Although this woman may have misinterpreted some of her doctor's comments, I have heard similar descriptions often enough to believe that even today women are actually being told such false horror stories.

In all fairness to doctors, the fact that some patients are not getting accurate information about VBAC is not because doctors intentionally try to deceive their patients. The fear of uterine rupture has traditionally been imprinted in the minds of American physicians even before they graduate from medical school. Remember that until recently statistics proving the safety of VBAC were not widely available.

These statistics are now available. A review of forty-three medical articles published over the past thirty-five years reveals that of the 11,027 women who have attempted vaginal birth after cesarean section, not a single woman has died due to uterine rupture.

We must remember that maternal mortality (the death of a woman relating to her pregnancy) is becoming rare in developed countries. Today, in the United States, only about one woman in 10,000 dies as a result of pregnancy, so the above statistics do not prove that there is absolutely no risk involved in VBAC. They do prove that the additional risk, if any, must be extremely small. To put the risk of dying from VBAC into perspective let's take a look at other causes of death. In 1983, 30,027 reproductive-aged women died from cancer; 13,354 women, ages fifteen to fifty-four, died of heart disease; 4,361 women in the same age group died of suicide; and another 3,480 women were murdered. Overall, 89,625 reproductive-aged women died in the United States during 1983. Of those deaths, not a single one was due to the supposedly treacherous VBAC!

In my comprehensive review of medical reports on more than eleven thousand women who have attempted VBAC over the past thirty-five years I have not been able to find a single report of a mother who has died due to the rupture of a low transverse uterine incision. It would probably be safe to conclude that driving on a freeway is riskier than natural birth after cesarean section.

What Is the Risk That My Uterus Will Rupture?

Countless women have been told that they shouldn't risk VBAC because their womb might rupture or "explode." The fear of uterine rupture goes back to the turn of the century when almost all cesareans were of the classical type and when uterine rupture was a very real problem. Today, the risk of serious uterine rupture is extremely low.

Doctors have had trouble agreeing on the definition of uterine rupture for a hundred years. We have used a hodge-podge of terms such as occult rupture, silent rupture, true rupture, symptomatic rupture, asymptomatic rupture, uterine dehiscence and uterine window when discussing the subject. Today many doctors have accepted a much more simple definition that divides uterine rupture into only two types.

Complete or true uterine rupture involves a tear that passes through the entire wall of the uterus. *Incomplete* uterine rupture involves a tear that does not go all the way through the wall of the uterus. The two types of uterine rupture have vastly different implications. Complete rupture can be very dangerous whereas incomplete rupture seems to have little or no significance for either the mother or the baby. In the past, some medical reports on uterine rupture lumped both types together, which made things very confusing.

Complete uterine rupture seems to be much less common than it used to be for several reasons. First, oxytocin (Pitocin), if needed, is used carefully to stimulate labor. When I was in medical school, the infusion pumps used today to carefully control the amount of oxytocin a woman receives were not used. The oxytocin was simply injected into the intravenous bottle and allowed to flow into the woman's arm. At times, large volumes of the medicine would flow into the woman's body, causing a massive cramping of the uterus called a tetanic contraction. It was also common practice to use oxytocin in the form of tablets that were placed in the mouth of a pregnant woman and allowed to dissolve. This practice resulted in an uncontrolled release rate of the medicine. The use of these tablets has been banned in the United States for several years. In any case, the injudicious use of oxytocin was responsible for many complete uterine ruptures.

Another reason for the decreasing incidence of complete uterine rupture has been the abandonment of some aggressive obstetric techniques. Difficult forceps deliveries and internal versions and extractions, methods that at times resulted in rupture of the uterus, are rarely done today. A final reason for the decrease in complete uterine ruptures is that classical cesarean sections are rarely performed today. It has been known for many years that the classical uterine incision has a serious risk of rupturing in subsequent pregnancies.

The exact incidence of complete rupture of a low transverse scar during an attempt at vaginal birth is unknown but all recent reports would indicate that the risk is extremely low. The best estimate is that this complication will occur less than 1 percent of the time. Perhaps more important, it seems that even when complete rupture of a low transverse scar does occur the consequences are not nearly as disastrous as those associated with complete rupture of a classical scar.

Incomplete uterine rupture is more common. Recent data show that perhaps 1 percent to 2 percent of women who attempt natural birth after cesarean section will have a partial separation of the uterine wall. Thus, 98 percent to 99 percent of women who attempt VBAC will have absolutely no problem with the uterine scar. The one or two women out of a hundred who do have an incomplete rupture, or asymptomatic dehiscence as some doctors call it, generally require no therapy. The thinned area of the uterine wall heals on its own and neither the mother nor the infant is harmed.

What Is the Risk That I Will Need a Hysterectomy?

Many women have told me that they've been warned that attempting VBAC is likely to result in a hysterectomy, which is simply not true. For many women, their cesarean baby was their first baby. Hence, if the VBAC resulted in a hysterectomy, it would mean that their second baby would be their last. For parents who strongly desire three or more children, the risk of hysterectomy and the irreversible sterilization that it implies is a serious concern. But the risk of hysterectomy resulting from a VBAC attempt is incredibly small.

There are two reasons why a hysterectomy might be required. Both are rare. The first is uncontrollable bleeding after the baby is born. This problem can happen to any woman whether she's had a previous cesarean or not. In fact, most emergency hysterectomies done for this reason involve women who have not had a previous cesarean. The second reason for hysterectomy is complete uterine rupture. As explained in the discussion of uterine rupture, it occurs in less than 1 percent of VBAC attempts. But even if a complete uterine rupture should occur, it does not necessarily mean that a hysterectomy will be required. More often than not, the defect in the uterine wall can be repaired in the same way that a cesarean incision is closed.

In 1985, doctors at the University of Southern California reported on the pregnancies of 1,209 patients with a history of previous cesarean section.[4] Of these women, 458 had elective repeat cesarean sections and 751 attempted natural birth. Five hysterectomies (1 percent) occurred among the 458 women who opted for elective repeat cesarean. Only two hysterectomies (0.2 percent) occurred among the 751 women who were attempting vaginal birth. Interestingly, neither of these were done because of uterine rupture. Both women had intact uterine scars and required the hysterectomy because of heavy bleeding, a complication that can occur regardless of whether or not a previous cesarean scar exists. Hence, of the seven hysterectomies, not a single one was a direct result of an attempted vaginal birth. In my own review of nine hospitals for the years 1984–1985, there were three complete ruptures out of 1,776

VBAC attempts. Of these, only one required hysterectomy because of uterine rupture.

The risk of hysterectomy resulting from VBAC attempt has been greatly exaggerated. Many of the old reports of hysterectomy were the result of rupture of classical uterine scars. Classical uterine incisions are rare today, and the old data are no longer valid. Even if we assume the risk of complete rupture of a low transverse incision to be 1 percent, and even if we assume that half of these wombs won't be repairable, the highest possible risk of hysterectomy we can project is 0.5 percent.

CHAPTER 5

Benefits of Natural Birth after Cesarean Section

What Are the Possible Benefits of VBAC for Me?

VBAC can benefit a woman in many ways—medically, psychologically, physiologically, and financially. Natural birth also benefits the baby, as will be discussed later.

MEDICAL BENEFITS

Prevention of death. When doctors discuss medical complications they usually divide their discussion into two areas: mortality and morbidity. In fact, most hospitals have weekly mortality and morbidity, or M&M, conferences. In simple terms, mortality means "death" and morbidity means "any problem short of death." The greatest possible benefit of

VBAC would be preventing the mother's death. Cesarean section is a major operation and, like all major operations, carries a risk of death.

Doctor J. R. Evrard reviewed statistics for Rhode Island from 1965 to 1975 and found that the risk of death associated with cesarean section was 26 times higher than with vaginal delivery.[1] Many doctors feel that this figure is an overestimate of the true risk of cesarean section. For example, Dr. Luella Klein, past president of the American College of Obstetrics and Gynecology, feels that a more realistic figure is the death of one mother per 1,000 cesareans.[2] Note that this figure is still several times higher than the risk of maternal death with a natural birth. In 1982, the Task Force on Cesarean Childbirth concluded that the risk of a mother dying as a result of a cesarean section complication was from two to four times higher than the risk of dying from a vaginal birth.[3]

A recent report on anesthesia-related maternal deaths in Michigan identified twelve women who died secondary to complications of anesthesia at the time of delivery.[4] Interestingly, eleven out of these twelve women died during or just after cesarean operations. Four of these women died due to complications of repeat cesarean section.

In any case, it's important to remember that the chance of a mother dying due to childbirth complications is extremely small. For vaginal birth the risk is 0.01 percent. Therefore, a doctor attending 200 births per year may never see a single maternal death.

Prevention of morbidity. Death, of course, is not the only possible complication of major surgery. Although the risk of death due to cesarean section is very small, the risk of lesser complications (morbidity) is quite high.[5] VBAC can reduce the risks of many of these potential surgical complications.

• *Prevention of infections.* Perhaps the most common complication of cesarean section is some type of postoperative infection. The three most common types of postoperative infections are endometritis, wound infections, and bladder infections.

Endometritis is an infection of the uterus (womb). About one-third of women who undergo a cesarean operation will develop a uterine infection. This percentage varies widely from one hospital to the next and, at some hospitals, more than 90 percent of women develop such infections after cesarean operations. The rate of such infections is lower in elective repeat cesarean sections, but not as low as for normal vaginal birth. In fact, infection of the womb after natural birth is rarely seen. A recent report estimated that when compared to vaginal birth the risk of uterine infection is five to ten times greater after cesarean section.[6] The same report noted that some hospitals have found the risk of lethal maternal infections to be eighty-one times greater after cesarean section than after vaginal birth.

Postoperative wound infection occurs in about 5 percent of cesarean section patients. When this complication occurs, the skin incision often splits open, exposing pus and infected tissue. The wound must then be cleaned and packed with gauze for a few weeks until the edges heal together.

Urinary tract infection (UTI) occurs in about 5 percent to 10 percent of cesarean section patients. This problem is often caused by the catheter that must be placed in the bladder during the cesarean operation.

When any infection occurs, intravenous antibiotics are generally administered until the fever resolves. This treatment often requires several extra days of hospitalization.

• *Prevention of blood loss.* The average blood loss at the time of a normal vaginal birth is about 600 milliliters (a little over a pint). In contrast, the average blood loss during an elective repeat cesarean section is about 1,000 milliliters (almost a quart). Hence, the blood loss with elective repeat cesarean section is almost twice the amount lost during a normal birth.[7]

• *Prevention of urinary tract injury.* Injuries to the bladder occur in about 0.6 percent of repeat cesarean sections and 0.2 percent of primary cesarean sections. This complication is three times more frequent in repeat operations because adhesions (internal scar tissue) often form after the first cesarean section, which makes the operation more difficult and increases the risk of cutting into the wrong type of tissues.

In addition to bladder injuries, on rare occasions (0.1 percent) the ureter, which is the tube that carries urine from the kidney to the bladder, will be injured. A recent report from a large university hospital revealed twenty-three bladder injuries that occurred during cesarean sections.[8] Ten of these injuries were associated with repeat cesarean operations. The same report also included seven patients with injury to the ureters. VBAC decreases these risks because in normal vaginal birth injuries to the bladder are much less common and injuries to the ureters never occur.

• *Prevention of bowel injury.* Accidental incision into the intestines at the time of cesarean section is quite rare. However, postoperative ileus, another complication involving the gastrointestinal tract, is not as unusual.[9] In this condition the bowels stop functioning and the intestinal contents tend to cause blockage. This condition often causes severe abdominal pain and vomiting. The treatment includes decompression of the intestine by inserting a suction tube down the patient's nose and into the stomach. Generally the condition resolves after a few days of stomach suctioning.

• *Prevention of blood clots in the legs.* Thrombophlebitis is a condition where blood clots develop inside of veins and block the circulation. The most common sites for these clots are the veins of the legs. The risk of thrombophlebitis is about ten times higher after cesarean section than after vaginal birth.[10] On rare occasions, pieces of these clots break off and flow into the lungs. This condition is called pulmonary embolism and it can be fatal.

• *Prevention of hysterectomy.* Many women have been warned that VBAC can result in uterine rupture. Many women have also been warned that such ruptures may lead to hysterectomy. But how many women are aware that multiple repeat cesarean sections can lead to hysterectomy? In 1952, doctors at Harvard Medical School reported on a rare condition called placenta previa accreta.[11] Placenta previa is a condition in which the placenta (afterbirth) is located so low in the uterus that it blocks the baby from being born naturally. Placenta accreta is a condition in which the placenta penetrates deeply into the wall of the uterus and cannot be removed after the baby is born. In placenta previa accreta both of these conditions occur.

The doctors from Harvard were intrigued that although cesarean section was uncommon in the 1940s, five out of nine cases occurred in women with prior cesarean operations. All nine women required hysterectomy and one of them died. Not much more was said about placenta previa accreta until 1985 when a fascinating report came out of the University of Southern California.[12] In this huge study it was found that placenta previa was found in only about one out of four hundred women if no prior cesarean had been performed. This finding was not very exciting since many other studies had shown the same thing. However, researchers also noted that in patients with one prior cesarean the risk of placenta previa was about one in 150, or about 2.5 times higher. Interestingly, the risk kept going up as the number of prior cesareans increased. For women with four or more prior cesareans, the risk of placenta previa was one in ten—forty times higher than for women with no prior cesarean!

Among the patients with placenta previa and no prior uterine surgery, only 5 percent also had placenta accreta. But for women with low placentas who also had a prior cesarean section, the risk of previa accreta increased fivefold to almost 25 percent. For women with two or more prior cesareans, the risk of a low-lying placenta (i.e., previa) being difficult or impossible to remove (i.e., accreta) was about 50 percent. In this study, eighty-two of the women with placenta previa accreta required emergency hysterectomies. Since both placenta previa and placenta previa accreta increased with increasing numbers of prior cesareans, the authors concluded, "The fact that the life-threatening condition continues to rise with multiple prior uterine incisions gives further support to attempted vaginal delivery after cesarean section."

PSYCHOLOGICAL BENEFITS

The possible psychological benefits of VBAC are much more difficult to determine. Depression is not uncommon in postoperative patients. The pain from the incisional site and the discomfort associated with gas pains and movement no doubt affect the psyche of every postoperative patient. As psychologist Dyanne Affonso noted in *Impact of Cesarean Childbirth*, women recovering from cesarean section often experience a feeling of inadequacy or loss.[13] The types of loss experienced by some women include:

- Concern about their inability to deliver vaginally, especially if childbirth preparation classes were taken.
- Loss of the ability to witness or participate in the birth.
- Loss of being allowed to have a significant person attend and participate as desired.
- Loss of control, or feeling a sense of powerlessness over the events surrounding the birth experience.
- Loss of, or interference with, the opportunity to immediately interact with the newborn baby. Loss of the immediate postpartum mother-infant bonding process.
- Feelings of inadequacy or loss of "womanliness" because of the inability to produce a baby in the "natural way."

- Feelings that parts of the birth process have been taken away.
- Longer loss from undertaking roles viewed as essential to the mother's self-concept, such as mothering the new baby, taking control of the household, and interacting with other children.

In addition to these feelings of loss, some women experience guilt for not being able to mother the new baby adequately. Successful VBAC might allow the woman to avoid these emotional problems.

PHYSIOLOGICAL BENEFITS

Today there is a renewed interest in the normal physiological function of breast-feeding. For women who choose to breast-feed, cesarean section can cause problems. Many women who deliver vaginally choose to breast-feed immediately after the birth. For the cesarean mother, even after the operation is over, breast-feeding will remain difficult, although it is possible. Obviously, cradling an eight-pound baby on top of an unhealed surgical incision will be uncomfortable.

FINANCIAL BENEFITS

It has been estimated that a cesarean section costs about $3,000 more than a natural birth.[14] Part of this expense relates to the cost of extra hospital days required to recover from major surgery. The costs of surgical supplies and operating room expenses are also contributing factors. For many women this cost seems unimportant since their medical insurance covers all or most of the bill. However, with the spiraling cost of medical care, insurance companies may no longer be willing to pay for the cost of unnecessary operations. If insurance companies decide not to pay for unindicated elective repeat cesarean sections, natural birth after cesarean section will result in the saving of several thousand dollars to the parents.

AVOIDANCE OF UNNECESSARY SURGERY

While it is true that many of today's surgical procedures produce miraculous results, the risks of major surgery must never be taken lightly. Among doctors there is often a lot of discussion about the relative merits of one type of operation as opposed to another. There are often several different operations, or modifications of operations, that will achieve the same goal. For example, there are literally dozens of surgical procedures that can be used to correct incontinence (the involuntary loss of urine). However, in their excitement over new and interesting types of surgical procedures, doctors often forget that the first decision, before deciding on what type of operation to perform, is to decide if *any* operation is really necessary.

There's an old saying, "If it's not broke, don't fix it." Today, some doctors have replaced this adage with new ones, such as "When in doubt, cut it out" or "A chance to cut is a chance to cure." Although these sayings are often stated in jest, they do reflect a changing attitude about major surgery. It is true that surgery is much safer today than it was fifty years ago. Developments such as powerful antibiotics and blood component transfusions have made once-treacherous operations very low risk. However, any operation can have major complications and, for that reason alone, the best operation will always be the one that can be safely avoided.

Does VBAC Offer Any Possible Benefits for My Baby?

Although most discussions about risks of cesarean section focus on maternal complications, the operation is not absolutely risk-free for the baby. VBAC can eliminate most of these risks.

Perhaps the most dangerous complication of elective repeat cesarean section, at least when considering the baby, is iatrogenic prematurity. Prematurity means that the baby was born too soon. Iatrogenic means that the problem was caused by the doctor. Hence, iatrogenic prematurity is generally used to describe a baby who was born too soon because of an error in choosing the date of an elective repeat cesarean section. This complication is very serious and sometimes fatal.

Since lung tissue is the last part of the fetus to mature, a baby born before its due date will often develop a condition called respiratory distress syndrome (RDS) or hyaline membrane disease (HMD). Babies with this condition often look totally normal at birth but begin to have problems breathing when they are only a few hours old. The baby will begin to flare its nostrils and make grunting sounds as it struggles to get enough air. The treatment often involves inserting a tube down the infant's throat and pumping air through a mechanical ventilator or respirator.

Usually another tube is inserted into the baby's umbilicus (belly button) to administer fluids and medicines that sustain the infant while the mechanical ventilator does its job. The newborn's lungs are very delicate and, despite the pediatrician's best efforts, the measures used to force air into the baby's lungs often result in another complication called pneumothorax. Pneumothorax is a rupture of one or both lungs that results in air leaking into the chest cavity. If this complication occurs, an incision must be made between the baby's ribs and a tube must be inserted into its chest. The chest tube then keeps the lungs from collapsing while the tube in the baby's throat pumps in oxygen.

Certainly the above description of a newborn infant impaled by numerous tubes and catheters does not paint a very pleasant picture. Even less pleasant is the fact that not all of these infants will survive. Others will survive with permanent disabilities. One way to prevent this type of prematurity is to perform an amniocentesis prior to an elective repeat cesarean section. Amniocentesis is performed by inserting a needle through the mother's abdominal wall and into the uterus. A small amount of amniotic fluid is then withdrawn and sent to the laboratory for analysis. If the test is positive it generally means that the baby's lungs are mature. Why don't doctors do an amniocentesis before every elective cesarean section? Amniocentesis is not without risk. A small percentage of the time the needle will cause damage to the placenta, baby, or the umbilical cord.

Although amniocentesis and meticulous calculation of due dates have reduced the incidence of doctor-caused prematurity, the problem still occurs. For example, in a study published in 1986, eight severe cases of iatrogenic prematurity were described.[15] These babies had no birth defects and would have apparently done well except for the fact that they were delivered too soon. Seven of these babies required mechanical ventilators (breathing machines) and four developed holes in their lungs (pneumothorax). One baby developed seizures (convulsions) and another baby eventually died. The only way to totally avoid iatrogenic prematurity is to await the onset of natural labor.

Another problem that seems to be related to elective repeat cesarean section is persistent pulmonary hypertension of the newborn. In this condition, the baby's lungs are apparently mature enough to function properly but for some reason they do not do so. In a study reported in 1985, twelve such cases were found to be related to elective repeat cesarean section at a single hospital.[16] Although only a few percent of babies were delivered by elective repeat cesarean section at the hospital studied, fully 17 percent of the cases of persistent pulmonary hypertension were found among these infants. All of these babies required mechanical ventilators and two of them died. In all fairness, I must point out that although these cases are worrisome, they do not conclusively prove that cesarean section increases the risk of persistent pulmonary hypertension in the newborn.

Some doctors believe that the process of natural birth is needed to squeeze fluid out of the depths of the baby's lungs. Cesarean section circumvents this process and may result in a less thorough drainage of lung fluid at the time of birth. There may be other beneficial effects of labor that we do not yet understand. For example, during thirty months at a single hospital in Indianapolis, forty-seven babies were admitted to the newborn intensive care unit suffering from respiratory distress after being delivered by elective repeat cesarean section.[17] All forty-seven babies required oxygen therapy. Several of these babies developed serious complications and one died. Interestingly, thirty of these babies seemed to have repiratory distress in spite of having apparently mature lungs. The doctors concluded that the respiratory distress in these thirty infants was due to their being delivered by elective repeat cesarean section.

Another hospital reported seventy-one cases of respiratory distress following elective repeat cesarean section.[18] Of these infants, 59 percent were considered to have been delivered too early. However, 41 percent were not delivered too early, but they developed respiratory distress anyway. It was concluded that "Infants born by elective repeat cesarean section, even those considered to be at 38 weeks or more of gestation, are at substantial risk of developing RDS."

Other fetal risks of elective cesarean section are uncommon but deserve mention. The baby's face could be cut by the scalpel when the uterine incision is made. Also, making a cesarean incision does not guarantee that the baby will slide out easily. Several medical reports have documented babies with broken bones that occurred during delivery through a cesarean incision. One unusual and upsetting episode occurred recently in which a doctor, while performing a cesarean section, accidently amputated several fingers from an infant's hand.

It should also be noted that at many hospitals elective repeat cesarean section is still performed under general anesthesia. Unfortunately, the medications used to put the mother to sleep invariably cross the placenta and can occasionally result in the delivery of an infant that is floppy and unresponsive. Although elective or routine repeat cesarean section generally results in the delivery of a healthy baby, the operation is not risk-free. Cesarean section can be dangerous and, on very rare occasions, fatal for your baby.

Does Cesarean Section Have Any Effect on Future Fertility?

Although it has not been proven, several studies have suggested that cesarean section appears to be associated with subsequent infertility. For example, in 1984, the New York State Department of Health followed up on more than 5,000 women whose first baby was delivered by cesarean section. [19] After five years, these cesarean mothers had 11 percent fewer babies than mothers whose first baby was born vaginally. A few months after this study appeared in the *American Journal of Obstetrics and Gynecology* an interesting letter to the editor was published.[20] Following is an excerpt from the letter:

> The study showing a decrease in future pregnancies among patients who undergo primary cesarean section probably comes as a surprise only to those who themselves have never undergone a major surgical procedure. . . . What may seem to a physician a relatively simple one-hour operation inflicts considerable anguish and suffering upon the one on whom it is performed. . . . Is it so remarkable that these patients

have no desire to undergo a repeated major abdominal operation with its attendant risks for themselves
and their infants? Would you?

Two more recent studies have looked at the issue of whether
or not cesarean section decreases future fertility. Doctors in
Finland confirmed that women who had their first child by
cesarean section had fewer second children.[21] In a similar
study, doctors at Cornell Medical Center also found a trend
toward infertility in women who had undergone the cesarean operation.[22]

Many women have been warned that attempting VBAC
can result in uterine rupture that may sometimes lead to
hysterectomy. This warning would be of great concern to
women interested in more children in the future. But, as
explained previously, multiple repeat cesarean sections may
actually be more likely to lead to hysterectomy than multiple VBACs! In any case, hysterectomy is a rare complication. The studies listed above indicate that there may be
other factors to consider when future fertility is discussed.
Since pelvic infections are a known cause for infertility,
and since such infections are much more common after
cesarean section than after vaginal birth, it certainly seems
plausible that cesarean section could lead to infertility. In
the past, some individuals have implied that VBAC could
be more hazardous to future fertility than repetitive cesarean operations. In reality, just the opposite may be true.

. . . .
CHAPTER 6
. . . .

Making the Decision

Should I Try to Have a VBAC?

Only the parents can make this decision. But there's a simple method that may help you make up your mind. This method can be used to help you make almost any complex decision. First, think of a balance scale. Mentally stack all of the benefits you might get out of VBAC on one side of the scale. On the other side of the scale stack all of the risks. Then ponder the scale for a while. Your goal is to decide if the benefits outweigh the risks. You can also look at the situation from the opposite point of view. You can stack all of the benefits of repeat cesarean section on one side of the scale and all of the risks of repeat cesarean on the other side. Again, your goal is to use all of the information you can gather to decide which way the scale tips.

At first this process may seem rather complicated, but if you give it a try you may find it quite helpful. At this point you may be thinking that it would be easier to just ask your doctor to make the decision for you. Unfortunately, if you don't make the decision yourself, you will probably be told to have a repeat operation. From the doctor's point of view, repeat operation means more money, less work, and less inconvenience. When faced with all of these factors, it's almost impossible for a doctor to offer an unbiased opinion.

Although I can't tell you what to do, I can tell you that in my hospital almost all women opt for VBAC. We strongly encourage all women with prior cesarean sections to attend our VBAC class. At a recent class there were nineteen couples. After weighing the risks against the benefits, eighteen of the couples chose to try for a natural birth. One couple is still deciding. Several of the women had difficult first labors but quite appropriately refused to believe that they were physically incapable of giving birth normally.

Has Anyone Attempted to Weigh the Risks Versus the Benefits?

Two very interesting medical reports have attempted to precisely weigh the risks and benefits of VBAC versus elective repeat cesarean section. Before we take a look at the results of these reports, let's take a minute to discuss how the comparisons were made. In the previous question we talked about using a hypothetical balance scale to help make difficult decisions. These two reports used a similar type of logic but in a much more intricate way. The technique used is called decision analysis.

The complicated statistical methods used in decision analysis are beyond the scope of this book, but basically the technique replaces the simple balance scale with complex flow diagrams called decision trees. Each branch point or node of the decision tree is like a separate balance scale. Once the decision tree has been constructed, its branch points are loaded with probability data. Calculations are then performed in order to meticulously evaluate the alternatives. With this basic picture in mind, let's take a look at what the two reports found.

The first report evaluated twenty thousand hypothetical pregnant women who had undergone cesarean section.[1] One group of ten thousand women were allowed to try for VBAC and another group of ten thousand women were delivered by elective repeat cesarean operation. The process of decision analysis uses known probabilities and statistics in an attempt to predict what would happen if twenty thousand women actually were to partake in such a study. What did the complex balance scale indicate? The analysis predicted 3.8 maternal deaths if all women tried for VBAC, but 4.6 maternal deaths if all women were delivered by elective cesarean section.

Surprisingly, thirty-seven more babies died in the elective repeat cesarean section group than in the VBAC group. It must be pointed out that the calculations assumed that a large number of babies would die from iatrogenic prematurity due to cesarean sections performed too soon. Today we can use amniocentesis to better evaluate fetal lung maturation prior to birth; thus, iatrogenic prematurity, although still a problem, is much less common than it was a few years ago. If we assume that all cases of babies being delivered too soon could have been eliminated, the number of babies lost in the elective cesarean section group would have been as low as the number lost in the VBAC group. In summary, this report indicated that the mortality risks for mothers and infants are no higher with VBAC than they are for repeat cesarean section.

The second report that attempts to weigh VBAC against elective cesarean section is even more interesting.[2] Whereas the first report looked mainly at the risk of mortality (deaths of mothers or babies), the second report looked at many other types of morbidity (complications short of death). Why is this important? Since the risk of mortality (death) is very low for either VBAC or elective cesarean section, a logical decision about which is safer must also weigh the risks of other possible complications (morbidity).

Among other complications, risk of uterine rupture, risk of hysterectomy, and risk of prolonged hospitalization were added into the decision analysis equation. This study even took into account such subjective nonmedical concerns as anxiety of awaiting labor, discomfort in labor, and disappointment of a failed trial of labor. What did this study conclude? After analysis of all the variables, it was concluded that "Trial of labor is superior to elective repeat cesarean section for both the mother and the neonate." It was further concluded that "In fact, to support the contention that elective repeat cesarean section and trial of labor are equivalent alternatives, one would need to artificially reduce the trial of labor success rate to less than 25 percent or increase the intrapartum risk for uterine rupture to greater than 20 percent."

Since the success rate for VBAC is 70 percent to 80 percent, and since the risk of uterine rupture is less than 1 percent, VBAC was clearly felt to be the better alternative in this report. In fact, the authors went on to state, "In regard to the case at hand, using simply utilitarianism, it should be argued that anything other than trial of labor after a previous cesarean section is *unethical* because the utility scores demonstrate that the trial of labor option holds the best outcome for both the individual patient and the patient population taken as a group."

As you attempt to come to a decision about VBAC, recall that reports from two major American university medical centers have attempted to weigh VBAC against elective repeat cesarean section. Both studies used the technique of decision analysis, which can be thought of as a series of statistical balance scales used to compare risks versus benefits. Both of these reports came out strongly in favor of VBAC.

What Does ACOG Say About VBAC?*

The American College of Obstetrics and Gynecology (ACOG) is the largest organization of Ob-Gyn specialists in the world. The majority of American obstetricians—about 25,000—belong to this medical society. One of ACOG's major functions is the continuing education of the nation's obstetricians. In fact, the first section of ACOG's bylaws states that its objective is to "foster and stimulate improvements in all aspects of the health care of women." To accomplish its goals, ACOG forms committees to continuously review current aspects of American obstetrical care. The results of these committee investigations and their recommendations are sent to the nation's obstetricians in a monthly ACOG newsletter.

In 1982, one year after the National Institutes of Health published a major report strongly in favor of VBAC, the prestigious American College of Obstetrics and Gynecology announced that vaginal birth was an "acceptable option" for women with a prior cesarean section. However, the original guidelines released by ACOG were so restrictive that few women would actually be allowed to attempt natural birth.[3] For example, it was recommended that in order to establish a VBAC program, a hospital should have an obstetric anesthesiologist in the hospital at all times. This recommendation automatically excluded almost every American hospital! Another restriction in the original guidelines was the recommendation that women with a prior cesarean section for "failure to progress" in labor not be allowed to attempt a vaginal birth. This guideline automatically excluded almost half of all women from attempting natural birth.

As more and more reports from all over the world substantiated the safety of VBAC, ACOG decided to revise

*For more information about the organizations discussed in this chapter, please see Appendix A.

its original guidelines. On January 25, 1985, the president of ACOG held a press conference to release the new revised guidelines[4] that include the following changes:

1. The restriction that VBACs be limited to certain major medical centers was lifted. ACOG's committee chairman, Fredric Frigoletto, M.D., explained that emergencies can arise during any labor. Since VBAC mothers are not at more risk of such emergencies than other mothers, any hospital that is not prepared to handle VBAC mothers should not be doing any obstetrics.

2. The original guidelines recommended that VBACs take place only in hospitals prepared to perform an emergency cesarean section within fifteen minutes. The new guidelines recommended that the hospital be capable of a response time of thirty minutes, which is the same as ACOG recommends for any laboring mother.

3. The restriction that an obstetric anesthesiologist be present in the hospital at all times was dropped.

4. The requirement that the obstetrician be physically present in the hospital during the entire labor was modified. The new wording stated that the physician should be "immediately available." This change is important since the old wording implied that even during a lengthy labor the doctor could not leave the hospital. It is a common practice for obstetricians to have their offices directly across the street from a hospital so that they can continue to see other patients while waiting for a woman to progress in early labor. The old guidelines would have required a doctor to cancel all appointments for the entire day every time a woman with a previous cesarean section was admitted to the hospital in early labor. For this reason alone many doctors found it difficult, if not impossible, to allow VBACs.

5. The original guidelines recommended against allowing labor in women whose first cesarean had been done because of failure to progress in labor. The revised guidelines pointed out that up to 70 percent of women who

fail to progress in their first labor will go on to have a successful vaginal birth if given another chance.
6. The revised guidelines pointed out that oxytocin, if required to augment labor, seems to have no greater risk in VBAC mothers than it does in the general population.
7. The revised guidelines stated that epidural anesthesia is not contraindicated in women with prior cesareans.

In October 1988, ACOG released the second revision of its original guidelines.[5] These new guidelines included the following major changes from the prior two versions:

1. By far the most dramatic change was in the recommendation that routine repeat cesarean section be eliminated. The 1984 guidelines had considered VBAC to be an option. Specifically, the 1984 guidelines stated that "The woman and her physician should discuss fully, early in the prenatal course, the option of a trial of labor." In contrast, 1988 guidelines stated that "The concept of routine repeat cesarean birth should be replaced by a specific indication for a subsequent abdominal delivery, and in the absence of a contraindication, a woman with a low transverse incision should be counseled and encouraged to attempt labor in her current pregnancy." Thus, as of 1988, ACOG was no longer recommending VBAC as an option, they were recommending it as routine practice.
2. The 1984 guidelines had excluded women with more than one prior cesarean section. In contrast, the 1988 guidelines stated that "A woman with two or more previous cesarean deliveries with low transverse incisions who wishes to attempt vaginal birth should not be discouraged from doing so in the absence of contraindications."

The entire text of ACOG's VBAC guidelines can be found in Appendix B at the end of this book. As you ponder your future childbearing options remember that ACOG, the world's largest organization of obstetricians, has strongly endorsed VBAC.

What Does ICEA Say About VBAC?

The International Childbirth Education Association (ICEA) is a nonprofit, primarily volunteer organization that was formed in 1960. ICEA has more than ten thousand individual members and three-hundred-fifty member groups in thirty-one countries. The organization's basic goal is to unite people who support family-centered maternity care and believe in freedom of choice based on knowledge of alternatives.

In 1980, ICEA published a document noting that cesarean section is a major surgical procedure, the use of which is "properly limited to those women in whom vaginal delivery cannot be accomplished without seriously jeopardizing fetal or maternal life and health."[6] In the event that a pregnant woman is told to have an elective repeat cesarean section, the ICEA Position Statement recommends that she "should undertake appropriate action to determine the possibility of a vaginal birth."

In 1987, the ICEA published a comprehensive review article on VBAC.[7] The ICEA review concluded that "The available literature indicates that morbidity and mortality for mothers and infants is less in carefully screened and monitored trials of labor than with elective repeat cesarean section."

What Does ASPO Say About VBAC?

ASPO/Lamaze is a nonprofit perinatal education organization composed of approximately 5,000 professional and parent members and an advocacy coalition of over 250,000 parent consumers who are members of "The Lamaze Family."[8] ASPO/Lamaze develops and promotes standards for childbirth education and family-centered maternity care, certifies Lamaze childbirth educators and publishes educational information for expectant and new parents. The *Lamaze Parents' Magazine* which is published by ASPO/Lamaze and is provided free to childbirth educators to distribute to expectant parents in Lamaze classes has a circulation of over 1.85 million and is read by over four times that many parents.

ASPO/Lamaze fully supports the guidelines of the American College of Obstetricians and Gynecologists: "Guidelines for Vaginal Delivery After a Previous Cesarean Birth." ASPO/Lamaze further asserts that unless contraindicated vaginal birth should be the expected and usual approach to childbirth following a previous cesarean birth because women usually experience fewer complications and VBAC is in most instances safer for both the mother and baby, the recovery period is faster, the financial costs are significantly less, and most important, it results in a more positive and satisfying childbirth experience.

ASPO/Lamaze believes that VBAC childbirth classes are important in preparing for a vaginal birth after a previous cesarean birth and that they should be available in every community. ASPO/Lamaze also believes that information on cesarean prevention should be an integral aspect of every Lamaze childbirth education course.

ASPO/Lamaze promotes VBAC by proving information on VBAC in its Childbirth Educator Certification Program, through continuing education programs for health professionals, and by providing information on VBAC to expectant parents through *Lamaze Parents' Magazine*. (Provided courtesy of Francine H. Nichols, RNC, Ph.D., president of ASPO/Lamaze.)

What Does AAP Say About VBAC?

In 1988, the American Academy of Pediatrics (AAP), in conjunction with the American College of Obstetricians and Gynecologists (ACOG), published a 356-page book entitled *Guidelines for Perinatal Care.*[9] The authors included some of the most prominent pediatricians and obstetricians in the United States. These authors concluded that "Unless there are specific contraindications to vaginal delivery, women with one previous cesarean delivery should be counseled to undergo labor in their current pregnancy." The book also concluded that "Data also show that maternal and perinatal mortality rates associated with vaginal delivery after cesarean delivery are no higher than those for repeat cesarean delivery."

What Does NIH Say About VBAC?

In the late 1970s, government officials became alarmed by the rapidly rising American cesarean section rate. They noted that the rate had tripled between 1968 and 1977. In 1979, the National Institutes of Health (NIH) organized a nineteen-member Task Force on Cesarean Childbirth. The task force, which included medical and nonmedical specialists from all over the country, spent the next year investigating the current status of cesarean section in the United States. The task force assembled at NIH headquarters in September 1980 to review its findings. The results of the task force investigation were published in 1981.[10]

The task force concluded that "Blood transfusions, endometritis, abdominal wound infections, thromboembolic phenomena, anesthetic complications, pyelonephritis, pneumonia, septicemia, and other measures of maternal morbidity are less common in the group with VBAC than in the repeat cesarean group." The NIH report clearly demonstrated that repeat cesarean sections were one of the major reasons for the rapidly rising cesarean section rate. After carefully investigating all available evidence, the NIH task force came out strongly in favor of VBAC.

What Does CPM Say About VBAC?

The Cesarean Prevention Movement (CPM) is an international nonprofit organization that was founded in 1982 by Esther Booth Zorn. CPM now has seventy-five chapters in thirty states as well as chapters in many foreign countries. Each year CPM counsels five thousand people through its main office and more than thirty thousand others through its local chapters.

For many years a major focus of CPM has been the promotion of VBAC and the avoidance of unnecessary repeat cesarean operations. The CPM cesarean fact statement explains, "Vaginal birth after cesarean (VBAC) is safer for both mother and infant, in most cases, than is routine repeat cesarean, which is major surgery." The document goes on to say, "Half of all cesarean women suffer complications and the maternal mortality rate for cesarean women is at least 4 times that of women with vaginal births."

The CPM philosophy revolves around the concept that birth is a normal physiological process and that with emotional support and education, the vast majority of women can deliver their babies as nature intended. A CPM brochure (*Working for the Birth You Want*) points out, "Many hospitals with lower cesarean section rates report better maternal and infant outcomes than do hospitals with higher cesarean rates. The number one reason for the increased cesarean rate is the outdated medical practice of doing repeat cesareans. The United States and Canada are the only countries in the world that do repeat cesareans routinely."

What Does C/SEC Say About VBAC?

Cesarean Support Education and Concern (C/SEC) is a nonprofit organization that was founded in 1973. One of this organization's main goals is to share information and

promote education on cesarean childbirth, cesarean prevention, and VBAC. C/SEC's Medical/Professional Advisory
Board includes professionals from the fields of obstetrics,
pediatrics, hospital administration, childbirth education, nursing, anesthesiology, psychiatry, and psychology.

I recently asked Beth Shearer, M.Ed., M.P.H., C.C.E.
(C/SEC's codirector) to comment on her organization's opin-
ions about VBAC. Her response was as follows:

> C/SEC has supported a woman's right to choose a
> vaginal birth after cesarean since its founding in 1973.
> When the first board of directors was formed in 1974,
> a third of its members had already had VBACs (though
> of course, we didn't use the acronym back then). The
> earliest issues of our newsletter, which began publica-
> tion in 1975, included birth stories from VBAC moth-
> ers. At that time, we were the only ones to take this
> position, except for a few lone clinicians. Every quar-
> terly newsletter since 1978 has included some men-
> tion of VBAC.
>
> In that year, we published a thorough review of
> the obstetrical literature, the first publication for par-
> ents about VBAC. After this point, we became much
> stronger advocates for VBAC, not just as an equal
> option with repeat cesarean, but as the preferable
> choice. This position was based on the total lack of
> evidence in the literature demonstrating repeat cesar-
> ean was safer. In the fall of 1978, we published a
> front-page editorial in our newsletter, titled "Where
> We Stand," in which we criticized the rising cesarean
> rate, and concluded, "One way to reduce the total
> number of cesareans being performed is to allow more
> women to attempt a vaginal delivery for a subsequent
> pregnancy. . . . Recent studies on vaginal delivery af-
> ter a cesarean have confirmed that the risk is low and
> the rate of success much higher than anticipated. We
> hope, then, that the now outdated dictum "Once a
> cesarean, always a cesarean" will be laid to rest. . . .

Indeed, we would like to see physicians take the initiative in suggesting this to women who are good candidates for vaginal delivery but who are unaware that it can safely be done."

Eleven years later this is still our hope, but not yet a reality. We believe there should no longer be controversy about VBAC. Simple common sense dictates it should be the standard of care. Elective repeat cesarean section is less safe for both mothers and infants. Major surgery should not be performed without evidence of benefit. A patient's fear, desire for convenience, or wish to avoid responsibility is not an adequate indication for major surgery. Women who have not had a previous cesarean are rarely allowed to choose a surgical delivery for these reasons. It is a double standard to allow women who have had prior cesareans to do so. It is even more inappropriate for women to undergo surgery based on physicians' convenience or fears. However, women need and deserve education about the safety of VBAC and how to cope with labor, attention to all their physical and emotional needs, constant one-to-one support during labor, and the chance to give birth with dignity and respect.

What Do Doctors in Other Countries Say About VBAC?

Although the policy of "Once a cesarean always a cesarean" has long prevailed in the United States, this belief has not been true in many other countries. In 1986, officials at the National Center for Health Statistics (NCHS) in Hyattsville, Maryland, sent out questionnaires to other countries to inquire about cesarean section statistics. The results of this survey were published in 1987 in the *New England Journal of Medicine*.[11]

NCHS found that cesarean section rates in the United States and Canada were about twice as high as the rates in other parts of the world. NCHS also found that in some countries the percentage of women having VBACs was eight times the American rate. For example, while the U.S. rate was about 5 percent, the rates in Scotland, Bavaria, and Norway were all around 40 percent. Only Canada, with 4 percent VBACs, ranked lower than the United States. NCHS looked at several factors that might account for the extremely high U.S. cesarean section rate. The NCHS report concluded that the largest difference between different countries in cesarean practice was in the percentage of women who had VBACs. Clearly, the American tradition of automatic repeat cesarean section has been a major factor in keeping its cesarean rate the highest in the world.

In contrast, VBAC has been popular in Europe for many years. Several medical reports in favor of VBAC came from the United Kingdom and Ireland during the 1950s and 1960s. More recently, favorable reports on VBAC have come from all over the world. Many of these reports are summarized in Appendix D at the end of this book.

One of the largest VBAC reports came from Ireland in 1987.[12] Of 2,176 women with previous cesarean section, only 395 (18 percent) were delivered by elective repeat cesarean section; 1,781 women attempted natural birth and 1,618 (91 percent) succeeded in avoiding surgery. Another recent report from Ireland points out that Irish obstetricians generally recommend VBAC instead of automatic repeat cesarean section.[13] There has never been a report of a maternal death in Ireland resulting from labor in the presence of a cesarean section-scarred uterus. The report also points out that while the U.S. cesarean section rate is approaching 25 percent, major hospitals in Ireland have rates ranging from 4 percent to 12 percent.

As noted above, Canada has had a policy of automatic repeat cesarean section similar to that found in the United States. However, in 1985, the Canadian National Consensus Conference on Aspects of Cesarean Birth came out strongly in favor of VBAC.[14]

Are There Special Classes for VBAC?

VBAC classes are becoming popular in cities all over the United States. Since almost a million cesarean sections are performed in this country each year, and since many of these operations are performed on women who desire more children in the future, there are millions of women who are potential candidates for VBAC. Unfortunately, not all of these women are fully aware of their options. VBAC classes should not be confused with childbirth preparation classes. Whereas childbirth preparation classes generally consist of a series of weekly sessions, a VBAC class is often a single meeting. During the meeting, topics such as those reviewed in this book are discussed.

You might ask, "If this book is intended to answer all of my questions about VBAC, why should I go to a VBAC class?" Probably the best reason is the opportunity you will be given to interact with other couples who have been though a cesarean section. Even if you choose not to say a word in the VBAC class, you may still get a lot out of the meeting by listening to what other people have to say. I'm not talking only about the information that will be presented by the instructor. You may find that questions and comments raised by other individuals in the class can be very helpful in your decision-making process.

An article entitled "Childbirth Classes for Couples Desiring VBAC" discusses different options for VBAC classes and suggests that prepared childbirth classes should be taken in addition to the VBAC class.[15]

How Much Research Has Been Done on VBAC?

If you choose VBAC instead of a repeat operation you will certainly not be sailing into uncharted waters. Since 1950, more than 50 detailed medical reports on VBAC have been published. At least three medical reports have been published on this subject each year for the past ten years. Few obstetrical options have been subjected to such careful scrutiny. These reports evaluated the labors of more than ten thousand women with previous cesarean sections. Without exception, each of these reports has supported the safety of natural birth after cesarean. More than 75 percent of the women studied in these reports were able to have successful vaginal births in spite of their previous surgery.

Thousands upon thousands of VBACs have been reviewed in detailed medical reports over the past forty years. The results of many of these reports will be summarized in the following pages. If you want more information about these studies, or if you'd like to read the actual publications, a complete list of these reports can be found in Appendixes C and D at the end of this book.

How Many Women Have Had VBAC?

As explained in the previous answer, medical reports have reviewed the labors of more than ten thousand VBAC mothers in meticulous detail. However, these reports represent only a fraction of the number of women who have actually given birth normally after a previous cesarean section. For example, a recent report from the National Center for Health Statistics estimated that twenty-one thousand American women gave birth by VBAC in 1985.[16] The same report estimated that fifty-three thousand women had successful vaginal births after cesarean section from 1980 to 1984. Thus, from 1980 to 1985, about seventy-four thousand American women had successful VBACs. Although more recent statistics are not yet available, VBAC is definitely becoming more popular in the United States and it is likely that at least 25,000 to 35,000 American women now have successful VBACs each year.

Thus, although automatic repeat cesarean section has

been very common in the United States, VBAC has certainly not gone untested. Extrapolation of the above statistics to include more recent data indicates that at least 250,000 American women have given birth by VBAC in the past ten years. Remember that these statistics only include VBACs that occur in the United States. In many other countries VBAC has been very common for decades.

What Are My Chances of Success?

As amazing as it may seem, your probability of a successful natural birth is almost the same as it is for woman who has never had a cesarean section. In 1982, Dr. Justin Lavin published a review of reports on VBAC for the previous thirty years.[17] Of 3,214 women attempting VBAC, 2,143 succeeded, which amounts to 67 percent. Remember that many of these statistics were collected years ago when many women had classical incisions. In 1985, I reviewed all of the medical reports published on VBAC during 1980 to 1984. I found that of 6,258 women who attempted VBAC, 5,356 succeeded and only 902 required a repeat cesarean, which means that 86 percent of these mothers were able to give birth normally despite their previous cesarean sections. Only 14 percent required a repeat cesarean.

As of 1987, the overall American cesarean section rate was about 25 percent. However, many of these operations (about 300,000 a year) are repeats. If we exclude all the repeat operations and look only at primary cesarean sections, the American rate is about 15 percent, which means that a woman with no prior cesarean section who enters an American hospital to have her baby has about a 15 percent chance of having a cesarean. As you may have noticed, this number is astoundingly close to the 14 percent found in the studies on VBAC mothers. Examination of these statistics can lead to only one logical conclusion: A woman with a previous cesarean section has about the same chance of successful natural birth as a woman with no previous cesarean!

Thus, we can conclude that the majority of women who attempt VBAC will succeed. This conclusion is true regardless of why the first operation was performed. It is true that women who had their cesarean section because of failure to progress in labor have a slightly lower success rate, but even these women will succeed in the majority of cases.

The discussion of "success" brings up a topic that deserves a little clarification. It is certainly true that many women have feelings of inadequacy or failure when labor ends with a cesarean section. I do not mean to perpetuate this concept, so let me clearly define what I mean by "success" in relation to VBAC. By "success," I mean only that the cesarean operation has been avoided. I do not mean to imply that a woman who ends up with a cesarean section has "failed." Essentially every medical report ever written about VBAC uses the term "success" when referring to vaginal birth. For logistical purposes this use makes sense. If I were to go through every chapter and change "success" to "labor after cesarean section culminating in a vaginal birth," this book would be much harder to read and about ten pages longer! So let's agree that in this case success means only that cesarean has been avoided.

CHAPTER 7

Pregnancy after Cesarean Section

Can I Do Anything to Increase my Chance of a Successful VBAC?

For one thing, don't have a ten-pound baby! There's no question that a large baby will cause a more difficult labor than a normal-size baby, which is true whether you've had a cesarean section before or not. Many women feel that they have no control over the size of their babies. They're wrong. It's true that a large woman with a large husband is very likely to have a large baby. But even this type of couple can, to some extent, control the birth weight of their child.

There is no question that the amount of weight you gain in you're pregnancy will influence the birth weight of your child. The average newborn will weigh about seven and a half pounds. Infants of mothers who gain too much weight will often weigh nine or even ten pounds. Giving birth to a ten-pound baby is generally not a pleasant experience regardless of whether you've had a prior cesarean!

How much weight should you gain? Most doctors agree that the optimal gain is about twenty-five to thirty pounds. Should this weight gain vary depending on how much you weighed before the pregnancy? Doctor Richard Naeye of Pennsylvania State University studied this question and found that women who are seriously underweight should gain thirty pounds whereas women who are seriously overweight should only gain about sixteen pounds. Although even experts disagree on exactly what is the safest pregnancy weight gain, no one recommends vast weight gains. I've seen several mothers attempt VBAC after gaining sixty or seventy pounds during their pregnancy. Most ended up with another cesarean operation. These comments are not meant to be critical of women who gain more weight than is recommended. Clearly, no two pregnant women have exactly the same metabolism. Many women who gain fifty or so pounds go on to deliver vaginally with no difficulties at all.

It's not only how much you eat that's important but what you eat. While a balanced diet is always a good idea, it's critical during pregnancy. Crash diets should never be the method used to control pregnancy weight gain. Books on optimal nutrition and exercise for pregnant women are available at most libraries and bookstores.

The above comments don't mean that mothers who gain a lot of weight or mothers with large babies shouldn't try for a natural birth. It's certainly true that even women who have had cesareans because their "pelvis was too small" go on to give birth to even larger babies than the one for which they had their cesarean section. But to increase your chance of success it is wise not to gain vast amounts of weight.

What are other factors that might increase your probability of having a successful natural birth? Finding a truly supportive doctor and educating yourself about what to expect in labor are two good ideas. Motivation is another important issue that can't be overemphasized. If you strongly desire a natural birth, and if you do not vacillate from this desire during your labor, your doctor will be motivated to respect your wishes. On the other hand, if you reach five centimeters and indicate that you'd like to "get things over with," many doctors will be quite happy to oblige. Remember that, for the doctor, performing a cesarean section involves less time and effort than attending to labor and natural birth.

Another thing you can do to increase your chance of success is to make sure that you discuss a few things with your doctor before you go into labor. You might want to ask your doctor if he or she has any special restrictions for VBAC mothers. For example, if your bag of water breaks before you go into labor (as it does 10 percent of the time), or if your labor slows down, will the doctor stimulate labor with oxytocin or insist on immediate repeat cesarean section? If you request pain medications or epidural anesthesia will they be allowed?

What If My Pelvic Bones Are Too Small?

Many women who attempt vaginal birth after cesarean section fear that they will undergo many hours of labor only to end up with another cesarean section because their baby is too large to fit through their pelvis. This fear is especially common among women whose first cesarean was done because their pelvis was supposedly "too small."

There are indeed women whose pelvic bones are too small to permit a vaginal birth, but such women are few and far between. Although almost one-half of primary cesarean sections are done for failure to progress in labor, small pelvic bones are rarely at fault. This fact is clearly proven since well over half of such women will go on to have successful vaginal births if they are given another chance.[1] Many times the VBAC baby will actually be larger than the baby that required the original cesarean section.[2] Although countless cesarean sections have been performed because of failure to progress, or because of cephalopelvic disproportion, very few women have truly abnormal pelvic bones. If you have had polio or a pelvic fracture, VBAC may not be for you. However, for the vast majority of women, normal birth is quite possible even with a fairly large baby.

Whether or not a baby will pass easily through the mother's pelvis involves more than the size of the pelvic opening and the size of the baby. One such factor is the way the baby's head is tipped as it comes through the pelvis. At times even a small baby will not pass easily through the pelvis if its head is tipped at an unusual angle.

It is true that large babies have a higher incidence of difficult births. For example, in babies weighing more than ten pounds it's common for the head to deliver with ease only to be followed by husky shoulders that get stuck. Shoulder dystocia can make the delivery very difficult. The American College of Obstetricians and Gynecologists VBAC guidelines include a precautionary statement about cases in which the baby's estimated weight is more than 4,000 grams (about 8¾ pounds). The problem with this statement is that it's impossible to weigh a baby until after it's born!

One might think that a doctor who examines pregnant women on a daily basis would be able to predict a baby's weight with great accuracy. Unfortunately this assumption is simply not true. Because each baby is surrounded by water, and because each mother's abdominal wall is different, it's almost impossible to accurately predict a baby's weight. When I was in medical school it was common to see friendly wagers made over estimated fetal weights. More often than not the inexperienced medical students out-guessed the obstetricians. Clearly, estimation of fetal weight is an inexact science.

Even new techniques like sonography (ultrasound) are far from perfect in guessing the weight of a term baby. Many medical studies have confirmed that as babies get larger ultrasound is less reliable in predicting their actual birth weight. For example, a group of doctors at Louisiana State University recently studied three sophisticated computerized ultrasound methods for determining fetal weight.[3] Surprisingly, they found that all three methods worked poorly for large infants. In some cases, the errors approached a full pound.

In another study the same group of doctors found that a very sophisticated ultrasound technique was able to correctly identify fifty-two out of fifty-eight large (8¾ pounds or greater) babies prior to birth. The problem was that the same technique also incorrectly labeled sixty-seven normal-size fetuses as being large. If the technique had been used to decide which women required cesarean section, sixty-seven women with normal-size babies would have been subjected to totally unnecessary operations.

So if a doctor decides not to allow women with apparently large babies to attempt VBAC, two errors are likely. The doctor may overestimate the baby's weight and end up doing an unnecessary repeat cesarean section, or the doctor may underestimate the baby's weight and allow labor with a baby actually weighing more than 8¾ pounds. Since the estimation of fetal weight is so subjective, an obstetrician who has little interest in VBAC might (perhaps subconsciously) overestimate the baby's size and recommend automatic repeat cesarean section. But what about the second error? Is it truly unreasonable to attempt vaginal birth even if the estimated fetal weight is more than 8¾ pounds? Probably not. I'll discuss why in the next question.

CASE HISTORY

Jamie is a twenty-six-year-old research assistant who had a cesarean section with her first pregnancy. Her physician had recommended x-rays of her pelvis when she was about a week away from her due date, since he felt that her pelvis might not be large enough for a vaginal birth. When she had the x-rays, her doctor believed that her pelvis was too small and scheduled a cesarean section before she went into labor. Her daughter weighed only six pounds three ounces.

"My daughter is nine years old, so I was very young when she was born. I had her in a small town in Oklahoma and she was delivered by my family doctor. I knew things had changed a

lot since then, that doctors didn't rely on x-rays very much anymore. I'd done a lot of reading about this and I really wondered if I couldn't have delivered my daughter normally. I never broke my pelvis or had a serious accident that might have made a normal birth impossible, and I've always been very healthy.

"When I became pregnant this time, I really didn't want another cesarean. I wanted to be able to have a baby the way it was meant to be had. I didn't think I'd feel satisfied until I at least had the experience of being in labor. Hopefully, I thought I would also be able to have a normal birth, but at least if I went into labor, I thought I'd be more fulfilled.

"I went into labor at 3:00 A.M. When I got to the hospital at 5:30 A.M. my contractions were very strong. I guess they really started out that way. I stayed home as long as I could stand it. When I told my husband that it was time to go to the hospital, he said, 'But honey, you've only been having contractions for two hours.' I guess the look on my face convinced him!

"My water broke just as I climbed into the hospital bed. The nurse checked me, told me that I was dilated to ten centimeters, and that I could start to push! I didn't believe her! When I asked her if she was sure, she just laughed and said that she'd been doing this for twenty years.

"Just at that moment I was overcome with this tremendous urge to push, so I got down to business. As it turned out, I pushed longer than the whole first stage of my labor. My doctor came in when I had been pushing for about an hour just to see how things were going. I was hard at work and convinced that I could do this thing.

"At two hours, I was exhausted and getting very discouraged. Dr. Blackstone examined me again and told me that the baby had moved down a lot into my birth canal, and that if I could just push a little longer, he thought it would all be over.

"This renewed my determination somewhat, but I felt I was really running out of steam. I tried everything to make the baby come faster. The nurse even helped me go into the bathroom and push on the commode a while. When I got back into bed, she moved a mirror over so that I could see what was happening as I pushed. After another half hour or so, I was able to see just a

little bit of dark hair on the top of my baby's head. What a sight! My husband and the nurse were cheering me on but I became so tired and could see for myself that the amount of hair visible just wasn't increasing.

"Dr. Blackstone came in again and was very happy with my progress. He said that he could see that I was very tired and that he thought he could place a little suction cup on the baby's head and help the baby out.

"I didn't have to think twice about that! The nurse got me into position in the birthing bed while my doctor was getting ready. He numbed me with a local and then warned me about the pressure I would feel as he was applying the vacuum device.

"With my next contraction I heard a whooshing sound and felt as though my insides were being pulled out. My husband was frantically trying to help me with my breathing but at that point I was beyond anything but a loud yelp.

"Just at that moment, my yell was drowned out by a louder cry, as my son, all eight pounds ten ounces of him, tested his lungs for the first time!"

What If I Have a Big Baby?

As discussed in the previous question, there are presently no reliable methods for predicting weights of large babies prior to birth. But let's assume that such a technique could be developed. Let's assume that such a test exists and you have just been told, by a very reliable estimate, that your baby weighs more than 8¾ pounds. Must you immediately opt for a repeat cesarean operation? I don't think so. Many individuals have interpreted the ACOG guidelines on VBAC as stating that labor should not be attempted if the estimated fetal weight is more than 8¾ pounds. However, a careful reading of the guidelines reveals that what is actually said is, "The effects of labor with an estimated fetal weight of more than 4,000 grams (8¾ pounds) has not been substantiated."

There are several recent medical studies that should

be of interest to any woman who would like to have a VBAC and suspects that she is carrying a large baby. In a 1984 report, doctors at the University of Southern California reviewed 140 women who had attempted VBACs with babies weighing more than 8¾ pounds.[4] Interestingly, 94 (67 percent) of these large babies were born vaginally, despite the fact that more than half of the women had previous cesareans for failure to progress. The authors concluded that there was no significant increase in risk with these large babies and that an attempt at vaginal birth was quite reasonable.

An even larger study reviewed VBACs in mothers with large (greater than 8¾ pounds) babies at nine California hospitals.[5] More than three hundred such cases were identified and more than half of these women delivered vaginally. There were no higher risks of complications in the VBAC mothers delivering large babies than in the VBAC mothers delivering normal-size babies. Perhaps even more importantly, there were no higher risks of complications in VBAC mothers with large babies than in mothers with large babies and no prior cesarean. In general, doctors don't recommend elective cesarean section for suspected large babies in women with no prior cesarean section. The California Multicenter VBAC report concluded that previous cesarean section mothers should not be treated differently.

It should be noted that when the mother has diabetes and a suspected large baby, or when the baby seems to be extremely large (more than ten pounds), cesarean section may be safer than vaginal birth.[6]

Finally, we must remember that although many women are concerned that their baby will be too large to be born naturally, statistics show that truly large babies are unusual.[7] For example, in 1983 there were 3,638,933 births in the United States. The average birth weight was seven pounds seven ounces. Only 9 percent of the babies weighed more than 8¾ pounds at birth. Hence, statistically speaking, the chances are only one out of ten that your baby will be in the vicinity of 8¾ pounds. If you carefully watch your diet the chances of having a normal-size baby will be even better.

What If I've Had Herpes?

The risks of herpes infections during vaginal deliveries have been blown out of proportion. It is true that on very rare occasions herpes can be dangerous or even fatal to a newborn. But while genital herpes is very common, the transmission of herpes from mother to baby is most unusual. Some recent estimates claim that 20 million to 50 million Americans have genital herpes. These figures would imply that between 10 and 25 percent of all Americans have herpes! This possibility is very difficult to believe. But even if we assume that only 2 percent of American women have recurrent herpes, this figure would mean that 72,000 births each year involve herpes-infected mothers. Yet there are only about 400 cases of herpes reported in newborns each year.

Because the risks of herpes seem to have been grossly overestimated, a vast number of unnecessary cesarean sections have been performed. A study in the state of Washington recently revealed that more than 50 percent of mothers with a history of herpes were being delivered by cesarean section.[8] With all these women headed for the operating room we have to stop and ask if these operations are harming more mothers than they are helping babies.

Current medical publications clearly point out that a history of herpes is not reason enough to perform a cesarean operation. Even a herpes outbreak that occurs during the pregnancy is not an indication to perform a cesarean section unless the lesion is present when labor starts. To rule out a minor herpes infection that cause no symptoms, cultures can be taken from the cervix every week during the last month of pregnancy. Most doctors, including myself, were taught that if these cultures are negative for herpes, there appears to be no reason for resorting to a cesarean operation, but if the cultures were not obtained, a cesarean section should be performed.

However, recent studies have demonstrated that it is

not necessary to obtain these cultures. In October 1988, the American College of Obstetricians and Gynecologists (ACOG) sent a notification to all 25,000 members stating that these cultures were no longer recommended.[9] The ACOG message concluded that cesarean section was only indicated if a herpes lesion was present in the vaginal area at the time of labor. The bulletin specifically stated that "Current knowledge indicates that routine surveillance cultures in pregnant women with herpes simplex virus (HSV) infections are of little clinical utility. In short, if there are no visible lesions, culture is not necessary, and vaginal delivery is acceptable."

CASE HISTORY

Sharon has a history of genital herpes. With her first pregnancy, five years ago, she had weekly cultures for the herpes virus during her last month. About three days before her due date, her physician called and told her that her last culture had been positive, although she had had no recent lesions. She had a cesarean section the next day.

"This time, I really wanted to have a vaginal birth, but at the same time, I wanted to do what was best for my baby. I didn't want to do anything that would harm him or her in any way.

"When I went to see Dr. Scott, she said that she had good news for me. Apparently, the recommendations for herpes in pregnancy had changed. She said that it was no longer felt to be necessary to do cultures for the virus. All the recent studies seem to show that the baby could be safely delivered vaginally, unless I had an outbreak close to the time I went into labor.

"At first I was skeptical about this. I brought my husband with me to my next visit, and we both had a long talk with Dr. Scott. She gave us some articles to read. After we both read the material, we felt better about the whole thing. I made up my mind that I would do it, that I would go for a VBAC.

"When I told this to Dr. Scott the next time I saw her, she was delighted with my decision. She told me that she would keep

her fingers crossed for me that I didn't have any lesions toward my due date and that we would check very carefully when I went into labor for any signs of an outbreak. Close to my due date, I was to let her know right away if I felt any of the tingling that I felt just before I broke out with a herpes sore.''

Six months later, Sharon went into labor at 3:00 A.M. At 6:00 A.M. she had a vaginal birth of a nine-pound son!

What If My First Cesarean Was Done Because of Fetal Distress?

Fetal distress means that the baby is in some kind of trouble and needs to be delivered immediately. Fortunately this event is rare and only a few cesareans out of a hundred are performed for this indication.

How do we tell if a baby is in trouble? The obvious answer is electronic fetal monitoring. But it's not that simple. Fetal monitors only test the baby's heart rate. To understand why this monitoring leaves something to be desired, let's imagine that the only tool your doctor has to evaluate adults is a machine called an "adult monitor." If you got sick, you'd go to the hospital and be placed in a small dark room with no windows and be attached to a machine which would measure how fast your heart was beating. The wires from this machine would go outside of your room to a monitor that would print out a continuous record of your heart rate. Now remember that this machine is not like an EKG; it could only check your pulse. It certainly couldn't test your blood pressure or measure your temperature. It couldn't test your blood or analyze your urine. It couldn't even tell if you're turning blue! Remember that the doctor can't even examine you; in fact, he can't ever see you!

How much could a doctor tell about your state of health by looking at this adult monitor? The answer is obvious: almost nothing. If the beat was slow you might be sick, but on the other hand, you might just be sleeping. If the beat was fast you might be in pain, but you might also just be moving around the room. Actually all the doctor could say *for sure* is that if your heart is beating you're alive!

Fetal monitors have no doubt saved the lives of many babies, but fetal monitoring is a very inexact science. We can't reach in and examine the baby, so we make the best of what we have. Unfortunately, even experts agree that at least half of the cesareans done because the baby's heart rate "looks bad" are unnecessary. The problem is we can't know for sure until the baby is delivered.

If your first cesarean was done because of fetal distress, you're probably fearful of labor. Your initial labor probably culminated in a shocking series of events. Your memories may include a frenzied ride to the operating room followed by an anesthesia mask being strapped over your face. If so, it's important to remember that fetal distress is generally not recurrent. Your chance of having fetal distress again is no higher than a woman whose first cesarean was for breech or herpes. Recent studies have shown that fetal distress will occur in only about 1.5 percent of VBAC attempts.[10]

Another study looked specifically at sixty-seven women whose first cesarean section had been performed because of fetal distress. In only two of these women (3 percent) did fetal distress recur during their next labor.[11] Hence, the chances that fetal distress will recur are extremely small and you're chances of having a successful VBAC are excellent.

CASE HISTORY

Sharon is a thirty-one-year-old bank executive who gave birth to her second child on Wednesday just before noon. The next morning, as she prepares to leave the hospital, she explains her feelings about what she has just experienced.

"I'll be honest with you, I really had doubts about going

through labor. The birth of my daughter was a nightmare. I remember that soon after I arrived at the hospital my doctor checked me and said I was only one centimeter dilated and that the baby did 'not look good' on the monitor. A few minutes later my baby's heart rate dropped and all hell broke loose. I clearly remember being rushed into the operating room thinking I was going to die. The last thing I remember was a smelly rubber mask being shoved over my face.

"After that experience I wasn't at all sure I wanted to try for a normal birth. I figured that if I was probably going to end up with a cesarean section anyway at least I could have one where everything was calm and well-planned. But I was told that the VBAC class was required for all women with prior cesareans regardless of how they felt about going through labor. So I went to the class even though I'd really already made up my mind against labor.

"The night I attended the class, there were several women present who came to talk about their VBACs. One of them had had an experience very similar to mine but had gone on to have a VBAC. I decided to give it a try but I certainly wasn't convinced that I'd make it.

"My contractions became very regular two days after my due date and when I arrived at the hospital just before midnight a nurse checked me and said I was only one centimeter dilated. I was sure that history was about to repeat itself. My husband tried to distract me but I couldn't take my eyes off the fetal monitor. I knew he was secretly as worried as I was since every time the machine skipped a beat he ran out to the nurses' station for help. The nurses kept saying the baby was fine but I kept thinking about what happened the first time.

"Most of the night my contractions were fairly mild and I was even able to get a few hours of sleep. By morning it was a different story. The doctor came in and checked me at 8:30 and said I was four centimeters dilated. I was excited about finally making some progress but the contractions were getting too strong. The doctor started to ask if I wanted some pain medication and I said yes before he even finished his sentence. The nurse gave me some Demerol, which made the contractions more bearable. At

10:20 I felt sick to my stomach. After I threw up the nurse checked me and said I was completely dilated. Those were the best words I'd heard in a long time. I pushed for just over an hour and then watched in a mirror as I gave birth to my son, Thomas. My husband couldn't believe the whole thing was happening. I'd never seen him so excited. He's usually the strong silent type but he cried as he cut the umbilical cord.''

What If My First Baby Was Breech?

If your first cesarean section was done because your baby was breech you have cause for celebration! The odds are overwhelming that you will not need another cesarean. Most studies on VBAC have shown very favorable results in mothers whose initial cesarean was performed because the baby was coming out buttocks or legs first. One such report revealed that 91 percent of 135 women whose cesarean section was performed because of a breech baby were able to give birth vaginally the next time.[12] I have personally reviewed the records of 456 women who attempted VBAC after an initial cesarean section for breech.[13] Of these women, 399 (88 percent) avoided a repeat cesarean operation and had successful VBACs.

Another obvious question that often comes up is "If I get pregnant again, what is the chance that the baby will be breech again?" The chance is very small. It is true that some women tend to have more than one breech baby, which may have to do with an abnormally shaped uterus. For example, some women have an extra piece of tissue inside of the uterus called a uterine septum. This wedge of tissue can keep the baby from rotating into the normal head-down position. If you have such a womb, the doctor who did your cesarean section probably would have mentioned it to you. If you're concerned about this, you can ask your doctor to review your operative report with you.

However, only 3 percent to 4 percent of babies are

breech at term. This fact is remarkable when one considers that early in pregnancy about half of all babies are breech. Why do the vast majority of babies flip into a head-down position? No one knows for sure. The important thing to remember is that even if your first baby was breech your chances are still nine out of ten that your next baby will be head-down. Even better news is the fact that your odds are also nine out of ten in favor of a successful natural birth.

What If My Skin Incision Is ''Up and Down''?

It makes absolutely no difference whether your skin incision is vertical or transverse. Remember that it is the uterine incision, not the skin incision, that determines the safety of attempting a natural birth.

Today, almost all cesarean operations begin with a transverse skin incision located along the pubic hairline, commonly called a "bikini" incision. In the past, a vertical skin incision, extending from just below the belly button to just above the pubic hairline, was often used. Some doctors still prefer this incision when speed is of the essence, for example, if the operation is being done on an emergency basis for fetal distress. Many doctors have found that the "bikini" incision can be done just as quickly. Since the up-and-down incision yields a cosmetically inferior result, and since it may not heal as well, most doctors have essentially abandoned its use in cesarean operations.

In any case, the important point is that the skin incision reveals nothing about the incision made in the uterus. Hence, it is not possible for a doctor to tell simply by looking at your skin scar whether or not you would be a candidate for a natural birth. Only the operative report, which explains how the uterus was opened, can answer this question.

CHAPTER 8

Labor after Cesarean Section

When Should I Call the Hospital?

Many women (and their husbands!) get extremely nervous as the due date approaches—this is especially true of first-time parents but it is also true of VBAC parents, many of whom have been erroneously told that they are in a very high-risk group. Although the risk of uterine rupture is quite low, it would probably be a reasonable precaution for VBAC mothers to come to the hospital a little sooner than mothers without prior uterine surgery. The only problem is that the longer a woman hangs around a hospital, the higher her chances of ending up with a cesarean section. I say this half in jest, but it is true that some childbirth instructors are now telling women to stay home as long as possible for this very reason. It is probably not a wise idea for VBAC mothers to stay home.

Many couples sit for hours timing contractions and they become frustrated when they can't determine whether true labor has begun. A good rule of thumb (at least near term) is that if your contractions are not truly uncomfortable you are probably not in labor. But remember that most hospitals have nurses who are specially trained to take calls from pregnant mothers. If you think you are going into labor, don't hesitate to call. Explain your symptoms and that you have had a previous cesarean section. The nurse will be able to guide you as to when you should leave for the hospital. Of course, if you break your bag of water or have any vaginal bleeding you should give the hospital or your doctor a call immediately.

Are Fetal Monitors Required?

If you've had a prior cesarean section, most obstetricians feel that fetal monitors are mandatory. I'm not among the fervent advocates of mandatory fetal monitoring in all women. However, it is true that medical studies have shown the value of fetal monitors in high-risk patients such as women with serious illnesses like diabetes or high blood pressure. No study has conclusively proven any benefits of fetal monitors in normal (low-risk) mothers. On the contrary, several studies have shown that electronic fetal monitoring has no value in low-risk mothers. Despite this fact, some hospitals now insist that every woman be monitored during her labor.

So, if I don't agree with the doctors who insist on fetal monitors for everyone, why do I insist on using the machines in VBAC mothers? Because, to the best of my knowledge, no baby has ever died due to complications of VBAC since fetal monitors have been used. I am aware of two babies that died due to rupture of a low transverse uterine incision, but both of these tragedies occurred many years ago, long before fetal monitors were available.

Although the chance that your previous cesarean will cause problems during labor is very small (less than 1 percent), the possibility does exist. In the rare event that your uterus does rupture, the fetal monitor might give a warning that could save your baby's life. For this reason, the monitors must be used even if you are healthy and are a low risk.

Do I Have to Have an IV?

I don't believe that there is any good data in the medical literature that can adequately answer this question. Since you've already had a cesarean section, and since this operation is never performed without an IV (intravenous), you're already familiar with IVs. To refresh your memory, an IV is a small plastic tube that is inserted into one of your veins. Why is this done? One reason is to slowly trickle fluids into the body in order to prevent dehydration. This procedure may be important if you are not allowed to sip fluids during labor. But the more important reason for having an IV is to assure that medications can be given rapidly if an emergency should arise.

To the best of my knowledge, most American doctors now recommend that an IV be placed in all laboring patients, not only women with previous cesareans. But, since no emergency will arise in the vast majority of labors, why do doctors insist on this procedure? When an IV is needed the most, it's often very difficult to insert. For example, if heavy bleeding occurs the veins tend to collapse, which can make starting an IV very challenging. In such rare situations, precious moments can be lost while time is spent trying to get an IV running.

The main disadvantages of an IV are that it is often quite painful (at least upon insertion) and that it tends to restrict the mother's movement. Our policy has been to insist upon IVs in VBAC mothers. However, if a woman strongly objects to an IV, I personally wouldn't press the issue. Again, this is my personal opinion; your doctor may not agree. Interestingly, the ACOG guidelines do not mention IVs.

Another alternative exists—a heparin lock—that might be a reasonable compromise if you feel strongly about not having an IV and your doctor disagrees. A heparin lock is a small tube, about the size of a paper clip with a tiny point, that is inserted into one of your arm veins and then capped. A drop of heparin (anticlotting medicine) is placed in the tube to prevent it from becoming plugged with clotted blood. There is no IV tubing connected to your body and no IV bottle hanging over the bed. If an emergency should arise, an IV tube can be quickly plugged into the heparin lock.

Must My Pubic Hair Be Shaved?

Some doctors have argued that it's better to shave the pubic hair of VBAC mothers so that time won't be wasted if an emergency cesarean section is required. But it has been shown that the chance of an emergency cesarean section is no higher in a VBAC mother than it is in any other mother.[1]

In any case, it only takes a few seconds to shave this area if the need arises. Since some women find the itching caused by hair regrowth to be very disconcerting, it is probably best to avoid unnecessary shaving of the pubic hair.

Do I Have to Have an Enema?

The most commonly known American obstetrics textbook states that "Early in labor, a cleansing enema is generally given to minimize subsequent contamination by feces which otherwise may be a problem, especially during delivery."[2]

However, I have not been able to find any scientific studies that document lower rates of postpartum infections in women who have had enemas. It would seem that the "contamination" is more an aesthetic issue than a medical one.

For some women, the passage of feces during the pushing stage of labor can be embarrassing. At times, this embarrassment may inhibit the mother's pushing efforts and possibly even prolong the labor. Hence, while enemas are not medically required during labor, and VBAC mothers are no exception to this rule, a reasonable approach would be to leave the decision about whether or not to have an enema up to the mother.

Must a Catheter Be Placed in My Bladder?

In the past, some doctors insisted that no woman with a previous cesarean section be allowed to labor without a tube being placed in her bladder. Today, however, most doctors agree that this procedure is totally unnecessary and perhaps even dangerous. In addition to being quite uncomfortable, the catheter itself causes a urinary tract infection in one out of every ten women.

As an intern I was reprimanded for allowing a woman to labor without a catheter. The woman thanked me, but an obstetrics professor dragged me over the coals. There were two reasons for the catheter rule. First, it was felt that if the uterus ruptured and the tear extended into the bladder, blood would appear in the urine and serve as an early warning sign. This reasoning did not make sense. After reviewing the records of literally thousands of VBACs, I've been unable to find a single case of the uterus rupturing into the bladder. Perhaps eighty years ago when classical (vertical) incisions were common the rule might have made sense. Today it does not.

The other reason given for insisting on catheter placement was that if a VBAC mother required emergency surgery, the tube would already be in place and thus valuable time would not be lost. This logic is also faulty. In the first place, a catheter could be inserted in a matter of seconds if an emergency arose. More important, the VBAC mother is at no higher risk of requiring emergency surgery than any other mother.

Can I Eat and Drink During Labor?

This subject is very controversial. Some doctors will allow no food or liquids during labor even in women with no prior cesarean. If a woman has recently eaten she faces a lethal threat in the event that she must be put to sleep (general anesthesia) for an emergency cesarean section. The danger is that while being put to sleep she could vomit and inhale the stomach contents into her lungs, which can result in a deadly condition called aspiration pneumonia. Almost half of all women who die in childbirth are killed by this complication.[3]

Ordinarily, when a person vomits there is no risk of this complication. An individual simply coughs up any vomit that accidently gets into the wind pipe. In fact, the body has an amazing automatic protective mechanism—the gag reflex—that prevents it from accidently inhaling food into the lungs. Since the wind pipe (trachea) and the food pipe (esophagus) sit side-by-side in the back of the throat, food occasionally "goes down the wrong way." When this happens, the violent coughing attack that ensues is often embarrassing, but it is also lifesaving.

The medicines used to induce general anesthesia have the unfortunate side effect of temporarily knocking out the lifesaving reflex. The same medicines can also cause nausea, which causes further trouble. First, the mother throws up, and then, unable to cough, she inhales the stomach contents down into her lungs. This occurrence is fatal more than 60 percent of the time.[4]

There are two reasons why aspiration pneumonia is so deadly. One is that when particles of food are inhaled into the lungs they block the small airways. The other is that when stomach acid is inhaled into the lungs it burns up the lung tissue. Avoiding food during labor will help to reduce the first risk but will do nothing to get rid of the stomach acid.

Rather than starve all laboring women many doctors now have adopted a reasonable compromise. Clear liquids such as water, ice chips, and fruit juices are allowed but solid foods are avoided in order to decrease the risk of aspiration of solid food particles should general anesthesia be required. To lessen the risk of stomach acid, some doctors recommend that women sip one ounce of antacid (milk of magnesia) every few hours during labor.

What about the VBAC mother? Many doctors allow the majority of their patients to drink liquids during labor but require that VBAC mothers remain strictly NPO ("nothing by mouth"). However, it must be remembered that the gag reflex works as well in VBAC mothers as it does in any other laboring woman. There is no risk of aspiration pneumonia unless general anesthesia is required. It has recently been shown that the risk of requiring an emergency cesarean section (and hence general anesthesia) is no higher in VBAC mothers than in other laboring women. Thus, VBAC mothers are at no greater risk for aspiration pneumonia than any other laboring women. Many doctors agree that it is reasonable to allow pregnant women to drink clear liquids during labor and there seems to be no logical reason for treating VBAC mothers any differently.

Can I Have Pain Medicine During Labor?

Although large amounts of narcotics administered during labor can cause problems with the newborn, most authorities agree that small doses can be of great benefit to the mother without in any way harming the infant. In the United States, most women request and receive some type of pain-relieving medication during labor. In contrast, the majority of VBAC mothers have been forced to endure labor with no such medication. While some women claim that the denial of analgesics is merely a method of discouraging natural birth after cesarean section, the matter is not that simple. The doctors' rationale for withholding pain killers was that the medicines might cover up the symptoms of uterine rupture. Pain "masking" may have been a logical reason for withholding analgesics thirty years ago when not much research had been done on natural birth after cesarean section and doctors did not know that the risk of uterine rupture was less than 1 percent.

In recent years, however, as dozens of medical reports have documented the safety of VBAC, the majority of doctors have lessened their restrictions and now offer VBAC mothers the same pain relievers that they would offer to any other laboring women. There is one glaring exception. Epidural analgesia, perhaps the most effective method of pain relief during labor, is still not offered to VBAC mothers in many hospitals. The epidural is similar to an older technique called spinal analgesia.

Both techniques involve injecting medication into the mother's back, but with a spinal the medicine actually enters the spinal canal and mixes with the spinal fluid. With an epidural the medicine is injected around the spinal canal but not actually into it. One advantage is that the excruciating spinal headache that often follows spinal analgesia is almost never seen with an epidural. Another advantage is that an epidural can provide pain relief for many hours whereas the spinal only lasts about an hour. With epidural analgesia the entire abdomen becomes numb and the contractions become much less painful. In some cases, the woman is totally unaware that she is having contractions. The epidural catheter is generally inserted by a specially trained anesthesiologist. Unfortunately, some hospitals do not have such a doctor and hence epidural analgesia is

not available. However, this method is becoming very popular and more and more hospitals are offering it.

Unfortunately, even at hospitals where the technique
is readily available it is often denied to VBAC mothers.
Prior to 1980, few medical reports mentioned the use of
epidural analgesia in VBAC mothers. However, from 1980
to 1984, ten different medical centers reported on this
subject.[5] A total of 647 women with previous cesarean
sections were given epidurals for pain relief during labor.
All 647 mothers and babies did well.

All recently reported data confirm that fear of masking
signs of uterine rupture is probably not a valid reason for
withholding pain relief from VBAC mothers. First, serious
rupture of a low transverse uterine scar is an extremely
uncommon event. Second, experience with thousands of
VBAC mothers has shown that pain is a very unreliable
sign of uterine rupture. For example, in 1971, an English
physician reported on a series of twenty repeat cesarean
sections performed because of severe abdominal pain that
seèmed to represent uterine rupture.[6] In nineteen of the
twenty women the previous scar was found to be totally
intact. Finally, a much more reliable sign of serious uterine
rupture is fetal distress noted on an electronic fetal heart
monitor. In the rare case of uterine rupture, this warning
sign would appear regardless of whether or not the mother
had been given pain relievers.

Today, most doctors offer conventional pain-relieving
medications during labor after a previous cesarean section.
However, the use of epidural analgesia in VBAC mothers
remains controversial. Although it may be premature to
conclude that epidural analgesia is totally risk-free after
previous cesarean section, we do know than during the
past several years medical reports have documented the
safe use of this technique in more than one thousand
VBAC mothers.

What If My First Labor Was Difficult?

Many women who have had a difficult labor that terminated in a cesarean section fear that they will have the same thing happen again if they attempt a normal birth. Although studies on VBAC generally do not directly address this issue, most such studies do report separate statistics for women whose cesarean section was performed because of failure to progress in labor or because of cephalopelvic disproportion. Many of these women had long and difficult first labors. Numerous medical reports have shown that even these women have a good chance of vaginal birth if they give it a try. See the question in chapter 7 regarding small pelvic bones.

Also remember that VBAC mothers do not have to endure labor without pain medications and that even epidural anesthesia is an option for VBAC mothers. A final point to consider is that while labor may be extremely unpleasant, it generally lasts only a matter of hours. After VBAC, most mothers are moving around the room almost immediately. In contrast, the postoperative pain associated with major surgery can last for many days.

Will Forceps Be Required?

They are used only on rare occasions. Forceps, large spoon-shaped metal instruments used to grasp the baby's head, are being used less and less. Thirty years ago, it was fairly common to pull a baby out with forceps as soon as its head could be reached. This procedure was especially used in VBAC mothers since it was felt that the last part of labor, the pushing stage, was too dangerous for the prior uterine scar. However, years of experience have shown that pushing or bearing down in labor does not put undue strain on the scar. The absolute proof of this fact is that even though the use of forceps in VBAC mothers has been virtually abandoned, uterine rupture remains a very rare event.

Although the use of these instruments rapidly declined in the United States, it should be noted that in some other countries the use of forceps to shorten the labor of VBAC mothers is still a common practice. For example, in a recent VBAC report from India, doctors stated that "To cut down the second stage of labor, 53.6 percent had forceps application."[7]

Is an Intrauterine Exam Necessary?

An intrauterine examination is given after the baby is born. The doctor puts his or her hand into the uterus and attempts to feel the previous cesarean section scar. Most studies on VBAC have included this procedure. Why? In theory, the doctor might be able to feel a small separation (dehiscence) or even a true rupture. However, there are several problems with this procedure.

First, after performing these examinations for several years I came to the conclusion that I didn't know any more after putting my hand inside the uterus than I did beforehand. Several times I felt areas that seemed to be in the approximate area of the old scar and seemed to be a bit thin. However, intrauterine examination is also occasionally required in women who haven't had a prior cesarean section. For example, if the placenta (afterbirth) doesn't come out completely the doctor may need to reach inside to remove any remaining fragments. On such occasions I made a point of carefully feeling the lower part of the uterus. Interestingly, I couldn't tell women who had a prior cesarean from those who had not. Even in women who had no prior surgery, I'd occasionally feel these apparently "weak" areas. Thus, the first problem with intrauterine examination for uterine scar evaluation is that it probably isn't very accurate.

Another problem with this examination is that its results appear to be meaningless! For example, suppose a doctor reaches inside you after a successful VBAC and feels what appears to be a thin area in the uterus. Several medical reports have pointed out that there is no need to do anything in this situation. If a small separation actually exists, it is almost certain that it will heal on its own with no therapy. My colleagues and I have seen dozens of women with apparent thin areas found after VBAC and none of these women have ever had to undergo surgery to repair them. Even if a suspicious area is found, there is no evidence that any treatment is indicated.

A third problem with this examination is that it involves blindly probing around inside the postpartum uterus. If a thin area does exist, there is at least a theoretical possibility that the examining fingers could poke through it and turn a nonexistent problem into a real one.

A fourth potential problem with intrauterine examination is that the examining fingers could carry germs into the uterus and cause a serious infection. This risk is probably very small but not nonexistent. Although doctors always wear sterile gloves during these examinations, germs are always present in the vagina and it is virtually certain that intrauterine examination carries some of these germs into the uterus.

A final problem with this examination is that it is not very pleasant. Since it would seem that this examination is of questionable validity, uncomfortable, and unlikely to provide any results that would alter your management, my opinion is that such an examination isn't worth performing. However, I can't take credit for coming up with this point of view. Some doctors had already abandoned this examination before I started medical school. For example, a VBAC report published in 1963 stated that "... nor are the patients examined vaginally following delivery to determine the state of the scar."[8]

It is true that the majority of medical research reports on VBAC have included this examination, because for statistical purposes the doctors are trying to determine the incidence of minor scar separations even if finding them won't change anything. In a nonresearch setting, the value of such examinations is questionable. The ACOG guidelines for VBAC do not mention any need for intrauterine examination.

It should be pointed out that everything I've said above presumes that you are not bleeding excessively. Although postpartum hemorrhage is fairly uncommon, any woman who has heavy bleeding after childbirth needs to be carefully examined and a VBAC mother is no exception.

There is one possible argument in favor of doing routine intrauterine examinations after VBAC. What if a "weak" area is felt in a woman who plans to have more children? Would this woman be at more risk of uterine rupture if she attempts more vaginal births in the future? Nobody knows the answer to this question. But it is reassuring that in the study from Ireland quoted above, many women had five or six vaginal births after cesarean section. No intrauterine examinations were performed and yet no uterine ruptures occurred in any subsequent pregnancies.

How Soon Can I Go Home After VBAC?

You can go home much sooner than if you have a repeat cesarean section! National statistics reveal that women who have repeat cesarean operations generally stay in the hospital three days longer than women who have VBACs.[9] In my study of nine hospitals in California, I found that VBAC mothers stayed in the hospital an average of just over two days while repeat cesarean section mothers stayed in the hospital an average of about four and a half days. At one hospital it was common for VBAC mothers to go home within twenty-four hours after giving birth.

The significance of an extra two or three days in the hospital becomes apparent when one realizes that the charges for mother and baby can exceed $1,000 per day! For young couples without adequate health insurance this situation can be a financial disaster.

Some women feel that the hospital might be a good place to stay and rest after having a baby. Years ago this belief used to be quite common, but it was probably never a very good idea. Hospitals are for sick people. New mothers and newborn babies are generally not sick. Because extensive utilization of antibiotics selects out resistant strains of germs, hospitals tend to spawn outbreaks of nosocomial (hospital-acquired) infections. An institution filled with seriously ill patients is probably not the best place for newborn babies to spend their first few days.

CASE HISTORY

Rosa didn't really want to have a VBAC; she wanted to have her second child by repeat cesarean. Her first child had been delivered by cesarean after a day and a half of a difficult labor, so it was reasonable to understand her reluctance to undergo a second labor. Her physician, however, told her that he did not believe in automatic repeat cesareans. He offered to refer Rosa to another physician if Rosa insisted on a scheduled cesarean. Because Rosa had been a patient of Dr. Matthews for years, and she really liked and respected her obstetrician, she decided that it was more important to have Dr. Matthews as her physician than it was to have a cesarean.

Rosa had two days of false labor before getting into the more active part of her labor. Her physician encouraged her to stay home until her contractions were close and strong. When she was finally admitted to the hospital, she had been having regular contractions for about three hours. Because of the two days of false labor, which had resulted in little sleep, she was already feeling exhausted. She was four centimeters dilated when she was examined for the first time. It was 9:00 A.M.

By 4:00 P.M. she was dilated only to seven centimeters, in spite of strong labor contractions. She felt that she couldn't go on, so she was begging for a repeat cesarean. Her obstetrician agreed, since she was making no progress in her labor.

Rosa was quickly prepared for surgery. Her abdomen was shaved just above the public bone and a Foley catheter was placed into her bladder to continuously drain the urine. She was moved to the operating room and placed on her side in preparation for the epidural anesthetic. Just as the anesthesiologist swabbed her back with an antiseptic solution, she had a tremendously strong contraction that also made her very nauseated. The nurse held Rosa's head as Rosa vomited into a small metal basin.

Suddenly, Rosa was overcome with a tremendous urge and began to involuntarily push with her contraction. The nurse grabbed a glove and after a quick vaginal examination announced that Rosa was completely dilated and that the baby was almost crowning!

Dr. Matthews was hurriedly summoned to the operating room, where at 4:47 P.M. he assisted Rosa with the birth of her son! The next day, when Dr. Matthews saw Rosa on rounds, she was beaming. At 10:00 A.M. she left the hospital, walking out with here son in her arms!

CHAPTER 9

Special Situations

What If I Go Past My Due Date?

The most important thing to remember about your due date is that it is only a guess. It's an educated guess but a guess nonetheless! The duration of the average human pregnancy is about thirty-eight weeks (266 days) from the time of conception. Note that I said *average*. Even if the exact day of conception is known, the date you will go into labor can't be predicted exactly. No two women are exactly alike.

In most cases, the exact date of your last ovulation (egg release) and the exact date that you conceived will not be known. For this reason, doctors estimate the due date by using a small calculator that counts ahead forty weeks from the first day of your last menstrual period. Since no two women ovulate exactly the same, and since even the same woman can ovulate on different dates from month to month, using the date of your last menstrual period may not be a very good way to predict when you will go into labor.

Modern technology such as ultrasound (sonogram) is helpful but still cannot predict the exact date of birth. Even the best ultrasound machine operated by a highly skilled technician or doctor can only guess the due date plus or minus about a week. Medical studies have shown that the most common reason for a baby being "overdue" is not that mother nature has made a mistake but rather that we have made a mistake in calculating the due date.

It is true that a few percent of women will go significantly past a due date that has been meticulously calculated. In these unusual cases, there seems to be something wrong with the biologic mechanism that causes the onset of labor. This unusual situation does put the baby at some risk and hence doctors have developed tests to evaluate the unborn child's condition. These tests include the nonstress test, the stress test, and ultrasound. Most doctors realize that the majority of babies who are "late" simply reflect the fact that the wrong due date was chosen. However, as a precaution they begin testing if the pregnancy goes one or two weeks past the supposed date. Note that going a few days past the predicted due date is very common and is not a reason for intervention or concern.

The nonstress test involves placing a device on the abdomen that records the baby's heartbeat. The stress test is similar except that contractions are induced while the baby is being monitored. An ultrasound machine is often used to check the baby's movement and the amount of amniotic fluid. What happens if one of these tests indicates that it would be better for the baby to be born rather than to wait any longer? If the mother has not had a previous cesarean the doctor will almost always recommend induction, which means getting the labor started. One way is to use a plastic device that is inserted through the cervix to create a small tear in the amniotic sac that surrounds the baby. This procedure, called rupturing the membranes, will cause labor to start in most women within one day. Another way to start labor is to use a medicine called oxytocin (Pitocin).

But what about the VBAC mother? While some doctors feel uncomfortable about using oxytocin on women with previous cesareans, more and more feel that it is safe and are treating their overdue VBAC mothers the same way they would treat their other pregnant patients. In the past few years, thousands of VBAC mothers have been treated with oxytocin with no major complications. However, inducing labor for women with previous cesarean sections remains controversial and even some doctors who strongly favor VBAC are against using oxytocin.

Oxytocin can be used to start labor or to help augment a labor that is already in progress. In the studies that I organized at nine California hospitals, we reviewed the records of 485 women who required oxytocin during their VBAC attempt.[1] We found that when oxytocin was used to augment labor (cervix open three centimeters or more), about 70 percent of the women delivered vaginally. This success rate wasn't much lower than for women who did not require oxytocin. However, when oxytocin was required to start labor, 53 percent delivered vaginally, implying that going two weeks past the due date and requiring oxytocin to start labor diminishes the chances of vaginal birth. Nevertheless, even in this unusual situation, it appears that the odds of a successful VBAC are favorable.

Perhaps the most important point of this discussion is that the most common reason for a baby not being born on time is that the wrong due date was predicted. As a precaution, fetal testing should begin when the pregnancy appears to have gone one or two weeks past the predicted due date. If these tests indicate a need for delivery, recent studies indicate that induction of labor is a reasonable alternative to automatic repeat cesarean section.

CASE HISTORY

Susan is a twenty-seven-year-old housewife, who has a three-year-old daughter delivered by cesarean section for fetal distress. In her postpartum room she relates the events of her recent birth.

"When my first baby was a week and a half overdue, my

doctor sent me to the hospital for a nonstress test to see if my baby was okay. When the nurse hooked me up to the fetal monitor, my baby's heartbeat dropped several times. The nurse notified my doctor, who came to the hospital immediately and recommended a cesarean section. He felt it would be best if we proceeded quickly, so I was given general anesthesia and was not able to be awake for my daughter's birth.

"It was rough afterward. I guess I did pretty well, actually, but it was hard having to take care of my daughter when my incision hurt so much. I think perhaps I didn't enjoy nursing as much as I might have in the beginning.

"Even with all this, I just expected to have another cesarean the next time I became pregnant. When I changed obstetricians with my second pregnancy, my new doctor, however, just assumed that I would have a vaginal birth this time! I was very anxious about trying for a VBAC. I kept having visions of being in labor for thirty-six hours and then ending up with another operation. So, I just thought it would be easier to have the cesarean again. I knew what that was like, but I didn't know what to expect from labor.

"But my doctor kept telling me that it would be better to have a normal birth. Every time I saw her, she would tell me something about the dangers of an automatic repeat operation. She said that with all the new stuff coming out about the benefits of VBAC, I should go for it. She also kept telling me that I really could do it. Slowly, I began to gain confidence and believe that maybe I could!

"My mother was very encouraging, too. She had three boys and two girls, all with easy labors, so she was convinced that I could deliver this one without any problems.

"My due date came and went. I was very apprehensive that the same thing would happen this time. My doctor reassured me that we would test the baby, and as long as the baby was okay, we would just wait. When I was a week overdue, I was scheduled for my first nonstress test. Imagine my relief when the baby passed it's test with flying colors! I had an appointment with my doctor two days later. On the morning of my visit I started having some contractions that were more like menstrual cramps

*and were not regular at all. When I was examined, I had
already dilated to two or three centimeters and my cervix was 100
percent effaced. My obstetrician decided that we should just go
ahead and induce labor, since I was a week and a half overdue
and my cervix was what she called 'very ripe.'*

"I called my husband to meet me at the hospital. He was
very excited that this would be the big day. At first, he hadn't
wanted me to try VBAC, but after going with me to my prenatal
visits a few times, he became convinced that it was the best way
to go. We both attended the VBAC class at the hospital where I
was going to give birth. This was very helpful in making him feel
more comfortable with my decision. The instructor addressed all
of our concerns and explained just exactly what would happen
when I was in labor.

"I arrived at the hospital shortly before noon, and was
comfortably settled with the fetal monitor attached and the IV
started when my husband arrived. My doctor appeared a little
later and gave instructions to start the Pitocin to induce my labor.
The fetal monitor showed that I was having some contractions
about every ten minutes, but I really didn't feel them very much.
An hour later, it was a different story!

"My contractions were coming every two or three minutes,
and seemed very strong to me. Little did I know how mild these
were compared with what was to come! My husband was helping
me concentrate on my breathing pattern, giving me ice chips, and
massaging my lower back. The contractions were so close he
didn't know what to do first.

"At 5:00 P.M. my doctor examined me, and cheerfully told
me that I was four centimeters dilated and that the baby had
moved down to a plus one station, well into my birth canal. She
broke my bag of water and inserted the internal monitors. An
hour later, I thought I was losing it. The contractions were so
intense that I couldn't relax, even in between. The nurse who
was with me suggested that a muscle relaxant might help, so
with my doctor's permission I was given a small amount of this
into my IV.

"I lost all track of time and place. My pains became more
and more intense, but at least I was able to relax a little. At 8:00

P.M. *I felt a strong desire to have a bowel movement. I frantically told the nurse that I just had to get out of bed and go to the bathroom. She smiled and said that she perhaps should examine me. Her eyes lit up when she did the exam. I was dilated to nine centimeters!*

"Forty minutes later, I just knew the baby was coming. My husband helped me get into position for pushing. At first, it was hard to know what to do, but I finally just surrendered to the forces within. After thirty-three minutes of pushing, my daughter was born! I couldn't believe that I had done it. It seemed so unreal that I had pushed this baby out of my body. Incidentally, she weighed just exactly the same as my first!

"I guess I'm really proud of myself. I never thought I could do it, but I guess this baby is proof enough. She's only twenty hours old and I feel like I could jog around the hospital!"

What If I've Never Had a Vaginal Birth?

If you're a bit nervous about attempting VBAC because you've never experienced a normal birth, let me enlighten you. You are not alone! The majority of women who attempt VBAC have never had a vaginal birth. One possible explanation is that the cesarean section rate is much higher in women having their first baby. Why this is true is a complex issue but it's definitely been proven. For example, a study from Case Western Reserve University in Cleveland, Ohio, revealed that a woman having her first baby was three times more likely to end up with a cesarean section than a woman who'd already given birth.[2]

In any case, it is true that most women who attempt vaginal birth after cesarean section have not had a previous vaginal birth. In a study of several California hospitals, I found that 1,181 out of 1,776 women attempting VBAC had only one prior baby, the one delivered by cesarean section. Thus, 66 percent of these women were trying for their first vaginal birth. Of these women, 861 (73 percent) had normal vaginal births in spite of the fact that they'd never done so in the past. It is true that women who had a normal birth prior to their cesarean section had a slightly higher chance of having a successful VBAC. However, the 73 percent success rate found in women trying for their first vaginal birth was not significantly different from the 74 percent success rate found among all women attempting VBAC.

What If My Labor Slows Down?

Since almost half of all primary cesarean sections are done because of failure to progress in labor, many women are concerned that the same thing might happen again if they attempt a vaginal birth. Before discussing what can be done about "slow" labor, we must first define "normal" labor.

Although no two labors are exactly alike, doctors have observed thousands of women and come up with some general rules. First, obstetricians usually divide labor into two parts. The latent phase, or early labor, begins when contractions get regular and ends when the cervix is about three centimeters dilated. (Doctors measure the cervical opening in centimeters. A centimeter is just under half an inch. The cervix spreads to about ten centimeters, or four inches, when it is completely open.) The duration of this part of labor is extremely variable. In some women, the latent phase may last only an hour or two, but it's also very common for the cervical opening to reach two or three centimeters (about an inch) and stay that way for several days. This occurrence is called prodromal labor and it is quite normal. Since this early part of labor can be prolonged even in normal women, many doctors agree that cesarean section for failure to progress is rarely if ever indicated before the cervix reaches three to four centimeters.

The second part of labor, the active phase, is when the cervix goes from about three centimeters to being completely open. This part of labor is more uniform. Generally the cervix will open at least one centimeter per hour.[3] Remember, however, that the examining fingers are not computerized micrometers! What one nurse or doctor calls seven centimeters another might call eight centimeters. Also remember that the one centimeter per hour rule is only an estimate.

If the active part of labor slows down, most doctors will recommend oxytocin (Pitocin) to stimulate the labor. However, many doctors are reluctant to use this medicine in women with prior cesareans. They fear that the medicine could overstimulate the uterus and cause it to rupture. This fear does not seem to be strongly supported by scientific evidence. When oxytocin is used as directed it causes contractions that are of the same intensity as spontaneous (natural) contractions. Dr. Edward Quilligan, co-editor of the *American Journal of Obstetrics and Gynecology*, has said that there is no reason to believe that a given pressure achieved by oxytocin is any more dangerous to a uterine scar than the same pressure achieved during natural labor.

A review of medical journals from 1950 to 1980 revealed that oxytocin was used in only about two hundred of the thousands of VBACs reported.[4] With the advent of fetal monitors many doctors began to feel more comfortable using oxytocin. A review of the medical literature from 1980 to 1984 revealed more than six hundred VBAC mothers treated with oxytocin.[5] In spite of the supposed risks involved, not a single baby was lost in any of these six hundred labors.

In a recent medical paper devoted specifically to the use of oxytocin in women with previous cesarean sections, Dr. Janet Horenstein and her colleagues conclude the following:

> Contrary to previous reports, the use of oxytocin in patients undergoing trial of labor with a prior cesarean delivery is not associated with an increased incidence of uterine rupture. On the basis of our experience, we

believe that oxytocin may be safely used in patients with a previous cesarean delivery who undergo a trial of labor. Oxytocin may be used for the usual obstetric indications in the patient with a prior cesarean birth provided that the labor and the fetus are closely monitored.[6]

I have been personally reviewing the records of all women attempting VBACs at eight large California hospitals for the past five years. So far, I've reviewed the records of more than five hundred women who were treated with oxytocin in spite of their previous cesarean section. Not a single mother or baby died in any of these labors. To be fair, it must be noted that there were two uterine ruptures in this group of women. Although these ruptures might indicate a trend toward slightly increased risk when oxytocin is used, they are not proof. In any case, the two women recovered quickly and both babies were healthy. We must also remember that although two wombs ruptured, almost five hundred did not. We found the risk of uterine rupture in women treated with oxytocin to be well under 1 percent.

A review of medical studies from all over the world (see Appendix D) reveals that oxytocin has now been used to treat thousands of VBAC mothers. Analysis of these statistics reveals that the risk of properly used oxytocin therapy is low. When dealing with women with no prior cesarean section, most doctors would not resort to cesarean section for failure to progress in labor without first trying to stimulate the labor with oxytocin. From the above data, it seems that it would be quite reasonable to treat VBAC mothers the same way. ACOG has reviewed the above studies and their revised VBAC guidelines now point out that the use of oxytocin in VBAC mothers seems to carry no greater risk than its use in the general population.

What If the Hospital Won't Allow VBAC?

To a hospital administrator, VBAC may not be a very appealing alternative to automatic repeat cesarean section. A hospital, just like any other corporation, must balance its financial books. Studies have shown that cesarean section mothers stay in the hospital an average of three days longer than VBAC mothers. When one considers that there are more than 300,000 elective repeat cesarean operations performed in the United States each year, the significance of these three extra days becomes obvious. The operating and recovery room charges generated by surgery do not hurt a hospital's financial balance sheet either.

There have been some cases where expectant parents and their doctor agree on VBAC, but the hospital administration may argue that the hospital is not prepared to deal with complications (such as having to do an immediate cesarean) that might arise during a VBAC attempt. This argument is not acceptable and you can easily prove it.

The only major risk of VBAC is complete uterine rupture. The risk of this complication is very small. It will happen to less than (perhaps far less than) one out of one hundred women attempting VBAC. However, there are many similarly severe problems that can arise during labor in women who have *not* had a previous cesarean. These include:

Complication	*Chance of Occurrence*
Placental abruption	1/100
(premature separation of the placenta)	
Placenta previa	1/200
(afterbirth blocking the birth canal)	
Fetal distress	1–5/100
(late decelerations and bradycardia)	
Breech or transverse lie	2–3/100
(in active labor)	
Prolapsed umbilical cord	1/100

Thus, there are many reasons why emergency surgery might have to be done during labor. Any one of these complications are as frequent as uterine rupture during a VBAC attempt; several are much more frequent. Hence, the chance that a VBAC candidate will require emergency surgery is, for all practical purposes, no higher than that of any other pregnant woman. This has now been documented in several medical reports. For example, doctors at the University of Texas found that less than 2 percent of VBAC mothers needed emergency cesareans during their labor, and that this figure was no higher than for mothers in labor without a uterine scar.[7] Another recent study found that less than 1 percent of VBAC mothers required an emergency delivery.[8] The bottom line is that any hospital that is not prepared to allow VBAC should not be doing obstetrics.

What If My Doctor Won't Allow VBAC?

In the past this problem has been a common one for parents interested in VBAC, especially those living in small towns. A survey of hospitals across the United States conducted in 1984 found that in very large hospitals (more than five thousand births per year) about 25 percent of women with prior cesarean sections attempted VBAC.[9] However, in the smallest hospitals (less than five hundred births per year) less than 2 percent of previous cesarean mothers attempted vaginal births. In the past few years, skyrocketing cesarean section rates have caused most hospitals to take a closer look at the indications for performing each cesarean operation. More and more small hospitals are now allowing VBAC as an alternative to automatic repeat cesarean section. In fact, some doctors feel so strongly that VBAC is safer than repeat cesarean section that they no longer perform any automatic repeat operations.[10]

In any case, let's assume that you've expressed interest in VBAC and your doctor says, "I only do repeat cesarean sections." You have two options: You can attempt to change the doctor's mind, or you can change doctors.

If your doctor says that he or she doesn't do VBACs, you might ask if you could be the first. Your doctor has probably already delivered hundreds, perhaps thousands, of babies. Your delivery will require no more skill or technical expertise just because you've had a prior cesarean section! Any doctor who is qualified to deliver a baby is qualified to deliver a VBAC baby.

If your doctor is accustomed to doing only repeat cesarean operations, and if you decide to try to change his or her mind, handle the situation tactfully. A doctor who has spent twelve years in premedical, medical, and postgraduate training may not take kindly to being told how to do his or her job. On the other hand, it's your pregnancy and it is only fair that you have some say about this important decision. Parents who express a sincere desire to experience a normal birth will be more likely to achieve their goal than parents who march in and demand a VBAC.

Finally, let's assume you have tactfully requested that your doctor reconsider his or her decision but that your doctor still insists on automatic repeat cesarean operation. Must you now give up all hope for a normal birth and prepare to head back to the operating room? Not necessarily. At this point, you might consider looking for another doctor. I didn't recommend this option first because it's an option that is not available to all pregnant women.

The statistics reveal that in small hospitals VBACs are least often allowed. Unfortunately, in these small hospitals there may be only a couple of doctors handling obstetrical cases. Since these doctors often cover night and weekend call for each other, it is unlikely that you could be guaranteed a trial of labor even if one of them agreed to it. Some women who strongly desire VBAC are willing to drive to the next town to achieve their goal. Most university hospitals now have active VBAC programs and such hospitals can be found in most major cities. If your doctor does not deliver VBAC patients, he or she may be able to help you find a doctor who does. I stress that the purpose of this book is not to foster hostility between you and your doctor, but rather to inform you of your options and to help you to achieve the type of birth that you desire.

CASE HISTORY

Casey is a thirty-nine-year-old costume designer who had her son by cesarean section when she was completely dilated.

"I still am not exactly sure why my son was delivered by cesarean. My labor was hard, but it had gone smoothly up to the pushing part. I was only in labor for seven hours total before the nurse told me I was all the way dilated. I had only pushed a few times when the doctor came in and told me he wanted to help the baby out. I guess I was kind of stunned by this but I didn't protest.

"They took me into the delivery room, where the anesthesiologist put in a spinal to numb me. The doctor put on forceps to help the baby out, but the baby just wouldn't budge. So, I ended up with an operation that I had never in my wildest dreams expected to have.

"The recovery was awful. I honestly think it was a year before I had recovered completely. I really enjoyed my son, but it was difficult taking care of him initially. Thank God I had lots of help, or I don't know how I would have managed.

"When I got pregnant again, I was determined not to have another cesarean. I talked to my doctor, who was aghast at the idea that I wanted to have a vaginal birth. I guess that I really hadn't wanted to go back to him after my first birth, but I didn't really know what to do at that point. I decided to call the nurse who had taught the childbirth education classes I had attended with my first pregnancy. She recommended that I get in touch with a local support group for cesarean mothers. They were able to give me a list of physicians in my area who did VBACs.

"I called one of the doctors on the list and made an appointment with him. During the visit, I got a feeling that he was only paying lip-service to the idea of VBAC, so I thanked him, left his office, and crossed him off the list. I was feeling slightly discour-

aged, but decided I'd better keep trying if I wanted to have my VBAC this time.

"Luckily, I hit pay dirt the next time. I found an obstetrician that both my husband and I felt was super. He was very supportive of our decision and told us up front that he was really committed to helping us have our VBAC.

"I went into labor right on my due date. The contractions started out more like menstrual cramps, but before long they were every three or four minutes apart. I had to call my husband at his office. When he rushed through the door a few minutes later, he took one look at me, grabbed the bag we already had packed, and practically carried me to the car!

"We had a van, so I stretched out in the back seat, trying to get into a comfortable position. The only thing that seemed to work was when I got on my hands and knees on the floor and did pelvic rocks with my contractions. I could tell that my husband was speeding, so I tried to tell him to slow down. He didn't listen but just kept barreling along.

"I could sense the relief in his voice when he told me that we were almost there. Just then, my water broke with a huge gush, all over the new carpet in the van! I didn't tell Jack that, because I was afraid he would kill us both if he drove any faster.

"Anyway, we got there in time. Dr. Frank didn't come to the hospital until the nurse called him and told him that I was nine centimeters dilated. He got there just in time to put on his gloves and catch my daughter. 'See,' he said. 'That's all you really needed me for. You did it all by yourself!'

"So, everything ended up just the way I wanted it. I'm glad I was persistent in finding a doctor who supported me in my desire for a VBAC. Now, if I can just find someone to clean the carpet in the van, I'll be all set!"

How Many VBACs Can I Have?

In the past, doctors have given two totally opposite answers to this question. Some claimed that each additional birth weakened the old scar and increased the risk of uterine rupture. In contrast, other doctors argued that each additional birth proved the strength of the previous scar. Neither group had any significant data to support their claims.

Today, with more and more women having VBACs, we're starting to see women coming back for a second or third VBAC. I've personally reviewed the records of about fifty such women and found no increase in risk. But even fifty cases is probably not enough to make a decision about the safety of multiple VBACs, so here's a look at what some other doctors have found.

A report from a major university hospital published in 1984 revealed that 96 out of 308 women who attempted VBAC had a history of at least one prior VBAC.[11] In fact, 3 of the women had given birth to five or more babies after their initial cesarean. These 96 women had no more risk of uterine rupture than the 212 women who had not had a prior VBAC. This preliminary evidence strongly suggests that subsequent pregnancies do not weaken a cesarean section scar.

A later report from the same hospital listed another 119 patients who attempted VBAC after a prior successful VBAC. Interestingly, this report revealed that the success rate among these women who had already had a VBAC was 96 percent.[12] This report seems to indicate that a successful VBAC significantly increases your chances of having another success if you decide to have another child.

A medical report from Ireland included some interesting statistics about women having several normal births after a cesarean section.[13] Out of 310 women with prior cesarean sections, 173 women had a first VBAC and 68 women had a second. This finding wasn't much different from what we see in American studies. However, 31 women had three normal births after an initial cesarean section, 18 women had four, 5 women had five, and 5 women had six. Finally, one woman had nine normal births after an initial cesarean section that had been performed for failure to progress in labor. Overall, 128 women had more than one vaginal birth after their initial cesarean section. There were no uterine ruptures in any of these women.

All available information indicates that multiple VBACs are as safe as, and may in fact be safer than, multiple cesarean sections. Parents considering large families would appear to be taking fewer risks by choosing multiple VBACs over multiple repeat cesarean sections.

CASE HISTORY

Sandy is a thirty-two-year-old registered nurse who is being seen for her first prenatal visit. This pregnancy is her fourth. Her first baby was delivered by cesarean section for a breech presentation. This will be her third VBAC!

"I'll never forget the time I went to my VBAC class with my second pregnancy. My son was only eleven months old, so the difficulty I had with the recovery from my first cesarean was still fresh in my mind. I had been in labor for six hours at home before I went to the hospital. When my husband and I arrived on labor and delivery and were examined by the nurse-midwife, she told us that the baby was coming buttocks first. We were rushed in for an emergency operation, since I was already dilated to eight centimeters. The recovery afterward was not easy, although I know I had what was considered a fairly 'uncomplicated postoperative course.'

"With my second pregnancy, I was so hopeful that this baby would not be breech, because I really wanted to have a vaginal birth. In preparation for this, I attended the hospital's VBAC class. I couldn't believe some of the other women in the class. They said they were only there because their doctor insisted that they attend. There were several who "just wanted to have another cesarean!" I tried to convince them that a vaginal birth was safer, but I'm not sure how successful I was.

"Sure enough my second child cooperated by staying in the head-down position through my whole pregnancy. So, here I am now planning my third VBAC. If only I could talk to some of those women again!"

What If I Have Twins?

Twins occur in about one out of one hundred pregnancies. If you used a fertility drug to get pregnant the possiblity of twins is much higher, perhaps one out of ten. There are two things to consider if you've had a previous cesarean and now have a twin pregnancy: first, how twins are generally delivered, and second, how your previous cesarean will change things.

In the past, doctors routinely allowed twins to be born vaginally to women with no prior cesarean, but this policy is rapidly changing. Several studies have shown that twin births are often complicated and that it's often the second (upper) twin that has serious problems. If you have twins, there are three ways the babies can be facing. About 50 percent of the time both babies will be head-down. This position is the safest and most doctors will allow a vaginal birth. Note that even when both heads are down, some doctors now recommend cesarean section.

About 25 percent of the time the first (lower) baby will be head-down but the second baby will be breech. In this case, some doctors try to turn the second baby to a head-down position after the first one delivers, but other doctors prefer to do a cesarean section. Finally, about 25 percent of the time the first baby will be breech. In this case, most doctors now recommend cesarean section regardless of how the upper baby is facing.

If you've had a prior cesarean section the vast majority of doctors will insist on a repeat cesarean. Doctors fear that the twin pregnancy will overstretch the uterus and increase the chance of rupture. Also, if the second baby is breech, most doctors won't try to turn it in a woman with a prior cesarean. (See the question dealing with breech babies.)

Doctors from Tacoma, Washington, recently reported on the successful VBAC of four sets of twins.[14] Although all four mothers and all eight babies did fine, the authors correctly concluded that "The successful trial of labor in four twin gestations does not constitute sufficient data to warrant any recommendation regarding VBAC."

A group of doctors in England reported on fifteen women with twins who attempted VBACs.[15] All fifteen women had successful vaginal births. The same doctors also listed information from other reports that included thirty additional women who had successful VBACs with twins. However, only about fifty cases of women attempting vaginal delivery of twins after a previous cesarean have been reported in medical journals. This is not enough data to adequately evaluate the safety of VBAC with twins.

What If My Baby Is Breech?

If you have had a previous cesarean section, and then in a subsequent pregnancy have a breech baby, what are your options? Note that whether the original cesarean section was done because of a previous breech baby or whether it was done for some other reason makes no difference in the context of this question.

First let's consider what a breech baby implies for a mother with no prior cesarean section and then we'll consider how your previous operation might change things. Many studies have shown that there is some increased danger with vaginal breech delivery. Hence, many doctors have decided to deliver all breech babies by cesarean section. Remember that we're not yet talking about women with prior cesarean sections but about *any* woman with a breech baby. National statistics indicate that 12 percent of American breech babies were delivered by cesarean section in 1970.[16] By 1978, this figure had increased to 60 percent, and by 1984, almost 80 percent of breech babies were delivered by cesarean section in the United States.

To avoid the dangers of delivering all these women by cesarean section, some doctors are now doing a technique called *version*, or more specifically, *external cephalic version*.

Version means that the doctor pushes on the mother's abdomen in an attempt to get the baby to flip around to the normal head-down position. Several recent studies have shown that about 60 percent to 70 percent of breech babies can be turned around by this method.[17] Although more data are needed before we can be absolutely sure, the technique seems to be safe.

Most studies on version have excluded women with previous cesarean sections. In 1969, Dr. James McGarry from Glasgow, Scotland, reported on 415 women with previous cesareans.[18] He stated that if breech babies were found, version was done just as if the woman did not have a previous cesarean. He felt that since the cesarean scar was strong enough to tolerate labor, it was also strong enough to tolerate the forces generated by turning the baby. There were apparently no complications; however, Dr. McGarry did not comment on how many women actually had breech babies and thus had this procedure performed.

In 1986, a group of doctors reported on version attempts in 158 women with breech babies.[19] 77 percent of the babies were successfully turned to a head-down position. The report mentioned that version was not attempted if the patient had a previous classical cesarean section, which implied that versions was allowed if a woman had a previous low transverse cesarean. However, in this report no information about the actual number of women with previous cesarean sections was given.

With the help of three of my colleagues I recently completed a study on this subject. The full results were published in the *American Journal of Obstetrics and Gynecology* in an article entitled "External cephalic version after previous cesarean section" (volume 165, August 1991). Briefly, here is what we found. There were 56 women with breech babies and prior cesarean sections who wanted to avoid another cesarean if possible. We were able to successfully turn the baby to the normal head-down position in 46 cases (82 percent). This success rate was just as high as it was for women with no history of a prior cesarean. There were no complications or problems. Clearly, these 56 cases aren't enough to absolutely prove that there is no risk to attempting to turn a baby if the mother has had a prior cesarean. But the results are quite reassuring and our opinion is that the additional risk, if any, must be quite small.

Since very few doctors will attempt to turn a breech baby in a mother with a prior cesarean section, the next question is, "Can't we simply leave the baby alone and allow a breech VBAC?" In the past, when vaginal breech delivery was considered routine, several reports on VBAC included breech births. In 1963, Dr. Allanbadia from Ireland reported twenty-two breech deliveries after previous cesarean and noted no complications. Although the statistics given above reveal that most breech babies in the United States are now delivered by cesarean section, some American medical centers still allow vaginal breech deliveries and a few will even allow them in women with previous cesarean section. For example, in the report from the University of Southern California mentioned above, thirteen women attempted breech VBAC and six succeeded. But such reports are few and far between.

In any case, it must be remembered that early in pregnancy almost half of all babies are breech (buttocks or feet-down). However, the majority of these babies will spontaneously turn to the normal head-down position by term. This has been proven by several medical studies. For example, by performing ultrasound examinations (sonograms) on 4,600 women who were seven months (32 weeks) pregnant, doctors in Sweden found 310 breech babies.[20] Over the next several weeks, 57 percent of these babies spontaneously turned to the normal head-down position with no help from the doctors. Only 3 percent to 4 percent of babies will remain breech at term. In properly selected cases, there may be a place for VBAC even if the baby can't be turned out of the breech position. However, since so few cases have been reported in the medical literature, there is very little objective data to support the safety of this alternative.

What If I've Had More Than One Cesarean Section?

A medical report that came out in 1982 reviewed the results of twenty-five VBAC studies published between 1950 and 1980. This report included statistics on more than 100 women with two or more previous cesarean sections who had been allowed to attempt vaginal delivery. (Refer to note 4.) The researchers found no serious problems and hence concluded that "There is little objective evidence to support the widely held view that multiple cesarean sections predispose to an increased risk of uterine rupture."

In 1985, I published a review of twenty-one VBAC studies from around the world that were published between 1980 and 1984. (Refer back to note 5.) I found three studies that included a total of about seventy women with more than one prior cesarean section. There seemed to be no increased risk associated with multiple prior cesarean sections.

The VBAC study I organized at nine California hospitals included eighty-nine women with two or more prior cesarean sections. These women seemed to do as well as women with only one prior cesarean section.

Doctors at the University of Southern California have recently reported the world's largest study of VBAC in women with two prior cesarean sections.[21] Of 501 such women, 69 percent delivered vaginally. The doctors concluded that "Trial of labor in patients with two prior cesarean deliveries appears to be a reasonable consideration and does not appear to expose the patient to unreasonable risk of harm." Over all, VBAC has now been reported in almost one thousand women after two or more previous cesarean sections. Although the numbers are not large enough to make any definite statements, it appears that the additional risk, if any, is minimal.

CASE HISTORY

Paula is a thirty-two-year-old dentist who had two cesarean sections, the first for failure to progress. She sits at home nursing her third child the day after its birth, talking to the registered nurse who is doing a follow-up home visit.

"I just knew that I could do it. I felt that my attitude had been all wrong with my first and second pregnancy. I never really had any confidence in my body to know what to do, so I was very frightened with each of my pregnancies. My first labor was a forty-eight-hour ordeal. I only dilated to three centimeters after twenty-four hours. When I arrived at the hospital, they broke my water and started to induce my labor shortly after that. In spite of strong labor and an epidural, I only dilated four more centimeters in the next twenty-four hours. By the time Dr. Jameson told me she thought I needed a cesarean, I was totally exhausted and willing to do anything to get the whole thing over.

"My recovery was not easy. I was not very interested in my baby for the first few days, but slowly things got better. It took me at least three months before I felt almost human again.

"I accidentally got pregnant when my son was six months old. In spite of the difficult time I had with the recovery from my first operation, I just knew that I wanted another cesarean. The thought of another forty-eight-hour labor was more than I could bear. My husband agreed with this decision.

"Dr. Jameson tried to talk me into having a vaginal birth, but I was adamant. No labor for me! Dr. Jameson reluctantly scheduled my cesarean for two weeks before my due date. This time, my recovery was much easier than before, although it still took me about four weeks to really feel back to normal again.

"When my second child was three years old, my husband and I started talking about having another one. We had agreed before we got married that we probably wanted four children. But with me having to have surgery each time, the likelihood that we would be able to have the family we wanted seemed remote. I just couldn't face the prospect of having two more major abdominal operations.

"So, I started thinking about what to do. I really wanted more children, but I felt like I couldn't go through with two more cesareans. While I was pondering my dilemma, my next-door neighbor became pregnant. She, too, had a cesarean with her first child. Was I ever amazed when she told me that she was going to have a natural birth this time. Hmm, I thought, we'll see about that!

"She and I had many conversations over the next seven months. She was so full of energy and enthusiasm about the idea of a vaginal birth. She would tell me about the visits to her doctor, the books she was reading, and the VBAC classes she was attending. I will have to admit that she inspired me to think that maybe I could try the same thing.

"Janet went into labor at 3:00 A.M. Her husband called to let us know that they were timing contractions, since I had agreed to watch her son when she went into labor. About 8:00 A.M. he called to say that he was bringing his son over to my house because he and Jan were leaving for the hospital.

"I was on pins and needles for the next several hours. When the phone rang shortly after four, I was hoping that it was news from Bob. Sure enough, but it was Jan, not Bob, on the phone. She was calling from her hospital room and was talking to me while she was getting her episiotomy stitched!

"Well, that did it! I decided right then and there that I was going to have the other two children that I wanted. When my husband came home from work that evening I told him about Jan's birth. I also told him about my determination to have a vaginal birth and that I wanted to try to get pregnant right away. He was most agreeable and suggested that we start trying that very night!

"I didn't get pregnant that night but it didn't take long before I had conceived. Dr. Jameson was amazed when I told her of my desire for a vaginal birth this time. She suggested that I might want to take a VBAC class to help allay some of my fears around labor. I read a great deal and did in fact attend a class when I was about seven months pregnant. During my pregnancy, I came to realize that part of my problem was due to lack of faith in my body's ability to birth a baby. I decided to seek counseling to help get more in touch with some of my fears and feelings about childbirth.

"I saw a wonderful psychologist who was very helpful to both me and my husband. By the time my labor started, I felt really ready for this wonderful challenge.

"I did need an epidural anesthetic when I was about five centimeters dilated, but I had made a decision beforehand that I would have an epidural again if I needed it. I was fully dilated one short hour after the epidural! Dr. Jameson told me that I could try to push, but that we would probably have to let the epidural wear off before I could really accomplish much.

"She left the room at that point. The nurse who was with me said, 'Come on, let's see what you can do.' I had been feeling somewhat of an urge to push, so with the next contraction, I gave it all I had.

"The nurse took one look and frantically started preparing the instrument table. Then she yelled over the intercom in the room, 'Dr. Jameson to Birth Room 3 stat!' Dr. Jameson came flying into the room with a puzzled look on her face. 'What's happening? Uh, oh. Guess I'd better hurry!'

"She didn't have time for her gown and mask, only her gloves. With the next push, my little girl came out with a whoosh, all wet and glistening. She was just beautiful and I was so proud.

"And, you know what? I didn't even need an episiotomy. 'Not even a skid mark,' Dr. Jameson chuckled as she took off her gloves."

What If I Want My Tubes Tied?

Since the average American woman will have only two children, and since any woman planning VBAC has already had at least one child, it is obvious that many women who are interested in VBAC will also be considering elective sterilization. In the past, many doctors have suggested that the best choice is to repeat the cesarean and simply tie the tubes at the same time. While this choice may be the best one for the doctor, it's not at all clear that it's the best choice for the mother.

Tying the tubes after a vaginal birth is a very simple procedure. The operation can be done through a tiny incision and the blood loss is usually less than one ounce. In contrast, the cesarean operation requires a huge incision and results in an average blood loss of about thirty-four ounces. This amount is about twice as much blood as is lost during a natural birth. Hence, performing a repeat cesarean section just because the mother wants her tubes tied results in the unnecessary loss of about seventeen ounces of blood. The additional blood loss is seldom mentioned to pregnant women when the options are presented. However, this loss is not trivial. Occasionally it results in the need for a blood transfusion and, as is fairly common knowledge today, transfusions have been linked to both hepatitis and AIDS.

What happens to women who request sterilization but have never had a cesarean? If it was indeed best to perform a cesarean section simply because sterilization was requested, then doctors would do the cesarean operation on any woman who wanted her tubes tied. But this procedure is never done. The doctor will allow a normal birth to occur and then will perform a simple sterilization procedure when the mother's condition is stable. I don't know of a single doctor who would recommend performing a cesarean section just because the mother wanted her tubes tied. However, if the woman has had a previous cesarean, many doctors will abruptly change their logic and recommend a repeat cesarean section.

What If My Water Breaks Before I Go into Labor?

In about one out of ten pregnant women the bag of water (membranes) will break before labor begins. Doctors call this occurrence premature rupture of the membranes. This event does not mean that the baby will be premature.

Actually premature rupture of the membranes means only that the bag of water has broken prematurely. To avoid any confusion, many doctors now use the phrase *preterm rupture of the membranes* to describe the rare situation in which the membranes actually rupture before the baby is mature.

For the membranes to rupture at term but before labor begins is a far more common situation. When this event occurs, many doctors recommend immediate induction (giving medicine to start labor), but there is strong evidence that doing so is totally unnecessary and may even be dangerous. In the first place, there is an 80 percent to 90 percent chance that labor will begin on its own within one day if the woman is just left alone![22] There's actually a 50 percent chance that contractions will start within twelve hours. Remember that breaking the bag of water is the most common method that doctors use to bring on labor. If the bag breaks on its own, the effect is still the same.

Doctors are concerned about the possibility of infection if the membranes remain ruptured too long before the baby is born. Certainly this concern is legitimate if the membranes have been ruptured for several days. However, the risk of infection from waiting twenty-four hours seems very minor. For example, one study of women with ruptured membranes found no increase in infections caused by waiting for the spontaneous onset of labor, but a threefold increase in cesarean section in women who had immediate induction of labor.[23]

Thus, for the woman with no prior cesarean section who has rupture of membranes before the onset of labor, the alternatives are either waiting for natural labor to begin or inducing labor with oxytocin. Note that I could find no medical reports that recommend resorting to immediate cesarean section.

Will your prior cesarean section change things? It is likely that your doctor will recommend immediate repeat cesarean section. One reason is that many doctors still feel uncomfortable about using oxytocin in women with prior cesarean sections. However, if your doctor will agree to simply leave you alone for twenty-four hours, the odds are that you will not need the medicine anyway. Remember that if nature is simply allowed to take its course, nine out of ten women will go into labor within one day after the bag of water breaks.

During the waiting interval it is best to avoid pelvic examinations since these can push bacteria into your uterus. It is also recommended that occasional fetal monitoring be used during the waiting period to assure that the baby is doing well. But if your doctor is strongly against waiting for the onset of labor, repeat cesarean section is still not mandatory. The medical literature strongly suggests that there is minimal risk associated with the proper use of oxytocin (Pitocin) in women with prior cesarean sections.

CASE HISTORY

Wendy is a thirty-five-year-old advertising executive who had her first child by cesarean four years ago. Her membranes ruptured and she did not go into labor. She was induced with Pitocin, but failed to dilate past two centimeters after ten hours, so a cesarean was performed. Wendy was determined to have a vaginal birth with her second pregnancy, but, unfortunately, history repeated itself and her membranes again ruptured before she was in labor.

"I was petrified that they would start the Pitocin and that I wouldn't dilate past two. But when the nurse-midwife saw me initially in the hospital, she explained that it might be best if we waited a while and let nature take its course. This was at about 6:00 A.M.

"They transferred me to a regular hospital room to wait for labor to start. I was allowed to walk around and drink juice and eat jello and stuff like that. I kept thinking that something would happen, that my labor would start, but no such luck. I think I fell asleep with my hand on my tummy feeling for a contraction.

"I was transferred back to labor and delivery the next day, and started with the induction of my labor. They said they didn't want to check my cervix yet because it might cause an infection. They put the monitor belts around my waist before they started

the Pitocin. When the midwife did examine me, I had been having fairly strong contractions for about six hours. Was I amazed when she told me that I was dilated to four centimeters and completely effaced! I looked at my husband and smack in the middle of a contraction I smiled just as big as could be. I knew then and there that I had gotten over the hurdle, that I could do it!''

Six hours later, after pushing for an hour and forty minutes, Wendy had an eight-pound thirteen-ounce daughter. Her husband helped deliver the baby's shoulders and cut the umbilical cord as the newborn infant lay on her mother's abdomen!

What If I Can't Get My Old Medical Records?

It's important that you get your medical records to find out what type of scar you have on your uterus. However, it is not necessary for you to obtain a complete copy of your medical records or your entire hospital chart, which could involve the copying of hundreds of unnecessary pages. What is necessary is a copy of your operative report.

The operative report is always typed and it is usually only one or two pages long. This document will almost always explain what type of uterine incision you had. The vast majority of operative reports will describe the uterine incision as low transverse, or low cervical. Rarely, it may say classical, or low vertical. As a precaution, it's a good idea to also request a copy of your discharge summary, because sometimes a doctor will forget to mention the type of uterine incision when he or she dictates the operative report.

But what if you can't get a copy of your operative report or your discharge summary? This problem should almost never happen. For both medical and legal reasons, hospitals tend to be very careful about keeping medical records for many years. But let's assume that you had your cesarean section in Afghanistan fourteen years ago and that the hospital, along with your entire medical record, was subsequently destroyed in a fire. This would mean that your type of uterine scar would be "unknown."

Does this mean that you are no longer a candidate for natural birth? Not necessarily. The issue of the "unknown" uterine scar type has been discussed in several recent medical reports. The University of Southern California School of Medicine probably has more experience with unknown scars than any other hospital in the world, because many of their pregnant patients have just arrived from Mexico, Central America, and South America. In 1984, they reported on 97 women who attempted VBAC with unknown type of uterine scar.[24] Eighty-seven percent of these women had successful vaginal births and there was not a higher incidence of complications in these mothers or babies when compared to women with documented low transverse uterine scars. The same hospital later reported on 592 women attempting VBAC with unknown uterine scar and found no increased risks. (Refer to note 8.)

If your medical records cannot be located, you may be able to make a reasonable prediction of your scar type by considering the following information. Today, the classical or vertical uterine incision is generally used only in very special circumstances. For example, if your cesarean section was performed because of placenta previa (afterbirth blocking the cervix), transverse lie (baby lying sideways), or a very premature baby (weighing only a few pounds), it is slightly more likely that you have a classical or low vertical scar on your womb. If your cesarean section was done for any other reason, such as failure to progress, failure to dilate, dystocia, slow labor, breech (near term), herpes, twins, or fetal distress, it is extremely likely that you had a common low transverse cesarean section. This type of incision began to replace the classical incision in 1926, and by the 1940s, some hospitals reported that less than 1 percent of cesareans involved the classical incision. National data for 1986 indicated that only about 1 percent of cesareans were of the classical type.[25]

What If I Had a Classical Cesarean Section?

Some doctors feel that a women with more than one prior cesarean section is a good candidate for VBAC, whereas other doctors disagree. However, almost all doctors agree that a woman with a prior classical cesarean section should not attempt VBAC. The actual risk of doing so is not known since almost all recent VBAC reports have excluded women with prior classical cesarean sections.

The low transverse uterine incision that is commonly used today is quite stable. Dozens of studies have shown that the risk of true rupture of a low transverse uterine scar is less than 1 percent. In contrast, studies done many years ago revealed that the classical scar will rupture about 2 percent of the time even before labor begins! If labor is allowed, the classical scar will rupture about 5 percent of the time.[26]

Not only is rupture more common with the classical type of scar but it is also more severe. In a review of twenty-five reports on VBAC from all over the world, Dr. Justin Lavin and his colleagues identified fourteen fetal deaths that were reportedly due to uterine rupture. Twelve of these fetal deaths occurred in women with previous classical uterine scars. Incidently, the two fetal deaths attributed to rupture of low transverse uterine scars both occurred more than twenty years ago, before the era of electronic fetal monitoring.

How Long Must I Wait after a Cesarean Section before Having a VBAC?

Rumor has it that it's safer to wait several years after a cesarean section before attempting a vaginal birth. There's absolutely no evidence for this belief. Studies on wound healing have shown that tissue regains the majority of its strength within a few weeks of an operation.

The tissue that gives a healing wound its strength is called collagen. According to a general surgery textbook, "Collagen content of the wound tissues rises rapidly between the sixth and the seventeenth days but increases very little after the seventeenth day and none at all after the forty-second day."[27] Since the uterine scar is almost fully healed within weeks after a cesarean section, there is no reason to postpone plans for having another baby.

What If I Change My Mind?

Since there are no statistics on this subject in medical books or journals, this question will be one of the few with a subjective answer. However, I have discussed this matter with at least a dozen other doctors, so what I'm about to say doesn't simply reflect my own opinion.

During labor all women are in some degree of discomfort and hence are likely to make decisions they might later regret. In fact, there are actually laws governing certain decisions during labor. For example, in California a woman cannot sign a surgical consent for sterilization within seventy-two hours of delivery. A woman upset with a difficult labor might request immediate postpartum sterilization. However, a few days later she might truly regret her decision.

It is also true that laws prohibit individuals from signing surgical consents for several hours after being treated with mind-altering drugs. Many women request pain-relieving medication during labor and these medications can blunt the decision-making process. A decision made under the influence of such medications might later be regretted.

I don't mean to imply that once a VBAC mother enters labor there's no turning back. Rather, it would seem reasonable for doctors to follow the same general guidelines for VBAC mothers as they follow for other women in labor. If a woman having her first baby began to have painful contractions and requested an immediate cesarean section, most doctors would certainly not rush her to the operating room. The proper course of action would be to carefully explain the course of normal labor and to offer support and pain-relieving medications. I believe that VBAC mothers should be treated the same way.

Some women are nervous about opting for VBAC because they feel that they won't be able to change their mind. In reality, many doctors are not excited about VBAC and would be quite happy to perform a repeat cesarean operation the moment a woman requests it. For this reason, it would be wise for you to thoroughly discuss this subject with your labor coach and your doctor before labor.

CASE HISTORY

Paula is a twenty-nine-year-old chemical engineer who is being seen for her annual exam and Pap smear. When her nurse practitioner asks about the scar on her abdomen, she relates that she had a cesarean section with her first pregnancy.

"I was in labor only about eight hours when I was dilated to ten. But then I pushed for three and a half hours and just couldn't get the baby out. With my second pregnancy I wanted to try to deliver my baby vaginally, but I was really afraid that the same situation would happen again. My doctor really encouraged me to have a VBAC, and my husband was gung-ho for the idea, too.

"I went into labor right on my due date the second time. The contractions started off with a bang! The first few were five minutes apart, and within half an hour or so they were coming every two minutes. We decided we had better head for the hospital, since we lived almost an hour away. On the way, my water broke all over the front seat!

"We checked in through the emergency room. The nurse there took one look at me, threw me into a wheelchair, and went flying down the hall to labor and delivery. I was barely able to

stand up to get into bed at this point. The OB nurse helped my husband plop me on the bed and undress me. When she examined me, she said 'Oh, I think it'll be a while yet. You're only dilated to three centimeters.'

"Well, I must tell you, I thought I was never going to make it. So, I started screaming that I wanted a cesarean and I wanted it now! I vaguely remember the nurse trying to reason with me, telling me that I really was doing very well. None of this penetrated. I just kept yelling, in between pant-blow breathing with the contractions, that I couldn't do this, that I wanted a cesarean, and I wanted it now.

"The nurse went to talk to my doctor. They both returned a few minutes later. My doctor tried to reassure me, but I was having none of it. Finally, I think he got a little exasperated with me, because he said something like, 'Being in pain is no reason to do a major operation!'

"Just at that moment, I was overcome with a tremendous urge to bear down. A quick examination showed that I was completely dilated and the baby was at a plus two station! I remember looking into Dr. Page's eyes and seeing what I thought was a gleam of triumph there.

"I got down to the business of pushing with a vengeance. Sure enough, twenty minutes later my daughter just seemed to pop out! When the nurse brought the scale in and weighed her, she weighed eight pounds and ten ounces, almost a whole pound bigger than my son!

"I was feeling slightly embarrassed that I had yelled so much, but at the same time proud that I had done it, that I had a VBAC. 'I did it!' I just had to yell one last time. As Dr. Page was stitching me up, I heard him mutter under his breath, 'I knew she didn't really want that C-section!' "

CHAPTER 10

Birth Alternatives

Can a Nurse-Midwife Attend a Birth After Cesarean?

Absolutely! First, let's clear up some confusion about midwives. A *lay midwife* is an individual who provides maternity care, may be licensed by the state, generally does not work in affiliation with a doctor, and generally has little or no medical training. Some lay midwives have had a great deal of experience, whereas others have had very little. In contrast, a *certified nurse-midwife (CNM)* is a licensed registered nurse who has taken special midwifery training and passed a national midwifery certification examination. Every certified nurse-midwife is affiliated with a physician who can be called upon if assistance is needed. Since I know quite a bit about certified nurse-midwives, but almost nothing about lay midwives, I'll confine my discussion to CNMs.

There are about two thousand certified nurse-midwives

in the United States. They deliver about 150,000 babies each year, or about 4 percent of American babies. Midwives generally give care to low-risk or "normal" pregnant women. However, VBAC mothers are not excluded. Numerous medical reports have revealed that VBAC is not associated with substantially more risk than any other childbirth.

Many certified nurse-midwives care for women with prior cesarean sections. In fact, at the hospitals with which I am affiliated, CNMs now provide care for the *majority* of VBAC mothers. I've reviewed the records of literally hundreds of VBAC mothers cared for by nurse–midwives and I've found the results to be excellent.

In an interesting article in the *Journal of Nurse-Midwifery*, six certified midwives are interviewed regarding how they would manage a patient with a previous cesarean section.[1] All agreed that they would recommend VBAC. The article concludes that "Vaginal birth after cesarean section is a safe and sensible option for a great many women."

Experts at most university hospitals now feel that VBAC is so safe that they include VBAC mothers in the low-risk group. By virtue of their training and experience, it would seem reasonable that nurse-midwives are qualified to care for VBAC mothers.

Can I Have a VBAC at Home?

From the first day of medical training, a modern obstetrician is programmed to believe that attempting a home birth is a dangerous and irresponsible act. To understand this situation, let's take a brief look at the history of home birth in this country. It may surprise you to learn that your own grandparents were probably born at home. In fact, at the turn of the century, the vast majority of American births took place at home. Less than 5 percent of American women delivered in hospitals in 1900. According to a textbook on the history of childbirth in the United States, "Nineteenth-century maternity hospitals were urban asylums for poor, homeless, or working-class married women who could not deliver at home."[2]

Of the forty-one American presidents, only a few were born in hospitals! President George Bush was born at home in 1924, on the second floor of a Victorian mansion outside Boston. But by the beginning of World War II, only half of all American births took place at home, and by 1983, 98.9 percent of all births took place in hospitals.[3] The justification for this mass migration from home to hospital is that the hospital supposedly offers safer births for both mothers and infants.

Fifty years ago about three babies out of one hundred died prior to reaching one month of age. Today, this number has been reduced to about one in one hundred. But to attribute all of this improvement to the elimination of home birth would be ludicrous. Many of the life-saving methods we take for granted today such as antibiotics and blood transfusions didn't exist fifty years ago. Today, in well-supervised home births, the risk to mother and baby is probably not extremely high. However, home birth is a very controversial issue. Many doctors, perhaps the majority, would like to see it declared totally illegal. The risk of VBAC is not substantially greater than the risk of any type of childbirth. However, since home birth is now discouraged by the overwhelming majority of American physicians, home birth after previous cesarean section cannot be recommended.

Although I am aware of many successful home VBACs, I would highly recommend that you do not consider it an option. VBAC mothers share one risk that sets them apart from other laboring women—the risk of uterine scar rupture. Although this risk has been vastly exaggerated, it is not nonexistent. While the risk is low, certainly less than one in a hundred, and although the tear is usually not serious, it must be remembered that on rare occasions such a tear can be dangerous.

Can I Have a "Natural" Childbirth?

I think it's fair to say that the answer to this question is "yes," although it would really depend on how you define "natural" childbirth. In the purest sense of the word, "natural" childbirth implies that the birth occurs as it would "in nature" with absolutely no medical intervention. Thus, to some individuals, a woman who has had even a small amount of pain medication at some point during her labor has not had a natural childbirth. To these people, a true "natural" birth could only occur at home with absolutely no medical intervention. At the other end of the spectrum are individuals who believe that anything short of a cesarean section is a "natural" childbirth, regardless of how many medical interventions have occurred, since the baby has been born via the "natural" passageway. Most people seem to agree that the true definition actually lies somewhere in between these two extremes.

To me, natural childbirth implies that a minimum amount of medical intervention has occurred. It also implies that the birth takes place in a natural-appearing setting rather than in a stark delivery room or operating room. Even within a modern hospital, rooms can be designed to look remarkably similar to cozy bedrooms. Medical equipment and supplies can be hidden where they remain out of sight unless they are actually needed. But a cozy bed and a rustic mural on the wall are not necessarily synonymous with natural birth. Natural childbirth also has to do with the way the laboring woman is treated by those around her. Is she perceived as a healthy woman about to have a baby or as a hospitalized patient in need of intensive care?

In the United States today, "natural" childbirth is a birth that occurs in a homelike setting, in the presence of supportive individuals, with medical interventions used only as necessary to assure safety for mother and child. I believe that this definition is fairly straightforward except that it brings up two more questions: "What is medical intervention and what constitutes the least amount of it?" With regard to labor and delivery, medical intervention includes a wide variety of instruments and procedures such as intravenous fluids, urinary catheters, pubic shaving, fetal monitors, and forceps. But exactly what constitutes the minimum amount of intervention is not an easy thing to define. Certainly a midwife attending home births and an obstetrician with a 40 percent cesarean section rate might strongly disagree!

However, after a great deal of deliberation, most doctors have come to the consensus that for the VBAC mother two interventions are required. These interventions are fetal monitoring and IV fluids. Many doctors now also agree that other interventions such as enemas, urinary catheters, pubic shaving, and prophylactic forceps delivery do not constitute necessary interventions.

It should be pointed out that the majority of American obstetricians now recommend (or require) that *all* women have fetal monitoring and IV fluids during labor. Hence, it's probably fair to conclude that in the context of modern American obstetrics the requirements of fetal monitoring and IV fluids for a VBAC mother do not imply that her childbirth will be any less natural than anyone else's. Interestingly, a recent report revealed that some individuals now allow VBAC mothers to labor with no fetal monitors and no IV.[4] In light of the discussion above, this practice cannot be recommended.

What About an Out-of-Hospital Birth Center?

Some doctors and a large percentage of midwives believe that it is difficult to achieve a truly natural birth setting within the walls of a hospital. However, many of these individuals also agree that home birth is not optimal. The out-of-hospital or "freestanding" birth center lies somewhere in between these two extremes. The birth center may actually be a home equipped with facilities to deal with minor emergencies. Birth centers generally have facilities available to transport the mother to a hospital immediately should the need arise.

At the present time, the issue of VBAC at an out-of-hospital birth center is a controversial one. In a book about birth centers published in 1986, it is stated that "VBACs are not eligible for freestanding birth centers."[5] However, some people obviously disagree since there are definitely some out-of-hospital birth centers that allow VBACs. The decision about whether birth centers are suitable places for VBACs comes down to the risk of VBAC compared to the risk of any other labor. It has been shown that the risk of requiring an emergency cesarean section is no greater during a VBAC than during any other labor. Nevertheless, one might argue that because of the small chance of uterine rupture it would be preferable for all VBAC mothers to give birth in hospitals.

However, the same argument could be made for other possible complications that are just as likely to occur in women with no prior cesarean section. Some examples would be premature separation of the placenta or prolapsed umbilical cord, which are both more common emergencies than rupture of the uterus. Women who choose to give birth in an out-of-hospital birth center should understand that such rare complications can occur and that they might have to be rushed to a hospital.

For women considering an out-of-hospital birth center, a very important question is, "How fast could you have a cesarean section if an emergency should arise?" The American College for Obstetricians and Gynecologists (ACOG) recommends that labor should take place where resources exist to perform an emergency cesarean section within thirty minutes from the time the decision is made until the procedure is begun.[6] Note that this recommendation applies to *all* mothers, not just to VBAC mothers. Out-of-hospital birth centers that can meet this requirement may represent a reasonable alternative for some VBAC couples. VBAC outside of a hospital setting is controversial, but if you are strongly opposed to a hospital birth, a free-standing birth center would be a far better alternative than a home birth.

What Is the Husband's Role in Birth After Cesarean?

In recent years, the husband's role in childbirth has increased markedly. When I was in medical school in the 1970s, fathers generally sat or paced in special waiting rooms during most of the labor. The mother-to-be was attended by a nurse part of the time and was left alone the rest of the time. As for the birth itself, I rarely saw a father in a delivery room. I can clearly remember trips to the waiting room to tell a man that he was a father. It was always exciting, but it also seemed rather strange that I should know before he did.

Today, at least in my area, it's unusual to see a woman in labor without her husband or significant other being present. One method of childbirth preparation, the Bradley method or Husband-Coached Childbirth, puts particular emphasis on the role of the husband. Many doctors and probably all midwives now believe in the importance of support during labor. Aside from the obvious benefits for the mother, many experts believe that the father's presence at the birth actually leads to a closer bonding between father and child.

These beliefs hold true for the VBAC couple. But there's one thing that's particularly important to remember about labor after a previous cesarean section. Other than the satisfaction of witnessing a natural birth, there's not much secondary gain for a doctor who attends a VBAC. In fact, as is discussed in detail elsewhere in this book, VBAC often means a lot more work (and perhaps less pay) for a doctor than a repeat operation. If a laboring woman starts requesting a cesarean section, it's likely that her doctor will offer moral support and a choice of pain medications. However, if that woman has had a previous cesarean section, the doctor may be sorely tempted to sharpen the knife.

This is where the husband may have a special role in VBAC. It's unreasonable to believe that a woman in labor can think as clearly as she could under normal circumstances. The same is true of any stressful situation. At some point during labor, especially during the pushing stage, it's not unusual for a woman to temporarily lose sight of her goals. Decisions made at such times could be decisions that would later be regretted. At such times an understanding and reassuring husband (or significant other) can mean the difference between another twenty minutes of pushing and another major operation.

Should I Take Childbirth Preparation Classes?

Absolutely. The best way to prepare for anything is to learn all you can about the subject in advance.

Taking a few classes will certainly not make you know more about childbirth than a doctor who has trained for many years. There are dozens of very rare complications that can occur during labor and these are the things doctors spend years learning to treat. But the majority of labors will be uncomplicated and childbirth classes will help you to clearly understand what normal labor and delivery is all about. Unfortunately, I've seen some women who arrive in early labor and don't have a clue as to what to expect. This lack of information always leads to a fear of the unknown.

There are several large organizations that train instructors to teach childbirth classes. The largest are the American Society of Psychoprophylaxis in Obstetrics (ASPO) and the International Childbirth Education Association (ICEA). Through childbirth classes you will learn conditioning and breathing techniques that can make labor much more tolerable. Note that childbirth preparation classes are not the same as VBAC classes, which are designed to meet the special needs of women who have had previous cesarean sections.

CHAPTER 11

VBAC—The Doctor's Dilemma

Do Doctors Prefer Cesareans over Normal Births?

In the past twenty years, literally hundreds of medical reports have discussed the impact of cesarean section on the mother and her baby. While these reports have presented detailed analyses of dozens of maternal and fetal implications of the operation, there's another topic that is almost never mentioned. What are the implications of cesarean section for the doctor?

In medical publications discussing the United States' rising cesarean section rate, objective factors such as breech, herpes, and fetal distress have been covered in great detail, but certain subjective factors such as doctors' personal feelings are seldom mentioned. Perhaps these are omitted because it seems to go without saying that the doctor will always exclude any personal considerations and base his or her decision (whether or not to operate) on what is best for the mother and her baby. This assumption is totally illogical. It presumes that doctors are superhuman creatures capable of totally excluding any personal feelings from their decision-making processes.

A few investigators are finally starting to take a look at this interesting subject. For example, a study of hospitals in Chicago proved that convenience does, in fact, play a role in doctors' decisions to perform cesarean operations.[1] The study was designed to look at the exact time of day when each cesarean section was performed at a major hospital. It was assumed that if the decision to perform each cesarean section was determined objectively, the same percentage of operations would be performed at all hours of the day. However, it was found that fewer cesarean sections were performed between midnight and 8:00 A.M. Another study recently confirmed this finding and found an excess of cesarean operations during the early evening hours.[2] Presumably this finding reflects the fact that some of the doctors used the cesarean operation more frequently at that time of day so they could go home and get some sleep. While these reports don't prove that any of the operations were unnecessary, they do strongly imply that subjective factors entered into the decision-making process.

Note that these two studies dealt mainly with women who had not had a prior cesarean section. When dealing with a woman who has had a previous cesarean, a doctor is faced with a much greater temptation. An automatic repeat cesarean section requires only about an hour of his time—an hour for which he will be richly rewarded. The positive implications of the cesarean operation for the doctor may explain, at least in part, why in spite of dozens of medical reports documenting the benefits of VBAC, the majority of obstetricians have continued to perform routine repeat operations. However, through years of personal and professional relationships with hundreds of doctors, I can honestly tell you that most physicians are devoted and caring individuals. They do, nevertheless, suffer from the same flaws and weaknesses as their patients. For the doctor, VBAC often means more work, more inconvenience, and less pay.

How Much Does the Operation Cost?

Having a cesarean section is substantially more expensive than having a normal birth. A doctor is almost always paid more for performing a cesarean section than for attending a normal birth. But this expense is only a small part of the total. A cesarean section is a major operation and consequently it requires a second physician to assist with the surgery. An anesthesiologist is also required as is an operating crew. The operating crew usually consists of a specially trained scrub nurse, a circulating nurse, and a recovery room nurse. Generally, a pediatrician or pediatric nurse is also present at the time of a cesarean operation. Hence, six or seven medical personnel are generally present for a cesarean section compared to only two for a normal birth. Of course, all of these extra doctors and nurses must be paid.

In addition to the extra personnel, there is often an operating room fee and a charge for the additional supplies necessary to perform the operation. But the major reason for the extra cost is the extra length of hospital stay. After a normal birth mothers usually go home in a day or two, but after a cesarean section most women stay in the hospital for four or five days. These extra days add up to big money. As of 1985, the average charge for one day in an American hospital ranged from a low of $559 in the Middle Atlantic states to a high of $907 in the Pacific states.[3]

It must also be remembered that the baby generally stays in the nursery as long as the cesarean mother is hospitalized. This results in an additional nursery fee that may be several hundred dollars a day. According to government statistics, the average total charge in 1986 was $2,620 for a normal birth and $4,330 for a cesarean section. This means that a cesarean section costs about $1,710 more than a normal birth. This estimate may actually be a bit low. According to the Health Insurance Association of America's 1985–1986 survey, the average cost (including doctor's fees) was $2,923 for a normal birth and $4,862 for an uncomplicated cesarean section.[4]

In a study I conducted in California in 1984, I reviewed hospital bills and found the average cost of a repeat cesarean section to be $5,101 compared with $2,087 for a VBAC.[5] The average repeat operation thus cost $3,014 more than a vaginal birth after cesarean section.

Do Doctors Get Paid More for Cesarean Sections?

Just because a cesarean section costs more than a normal birth, it doesn't mean that all of the extra money goes to the doctor. In fact, most of the extra money goes to the hospital. How much actually goes to the doctor? A survey of doctors in one area of California found that the average charge for prenatal care and normal vaginal delivery was $1,662. The average charge for the same amount of prenatal care but with cesarean section delivery was $2,230.

Who Pays for a Cesarean Operation?

As discussed in the previous questions, a cesarean operation costs about $2,000 to $3,000 more than a normal vaginal birth. Unfortunately, not all pregnant woman have adequate health insurance. In fact, about 35 million Americans don't have any health insurance at all. An additional five million American women have insurance policies that don't cover maternity care. A large number of women are covered under their husband's health insurance policy. If the husband changes jobs during the pregnancy it is quite possible that the new employer will consider the pregnancy to be a "preexisting condition." In this case, maternity costs may not be covered.

Most women give birth when they are in their twenties or early thirties and have minimal financial resources. In 1984, for example, the average young couple had a combined annual family income of under $20,000. The cost of having a baby can easily add up to 25 percent of a young couple's annual after-tax income. The additional cost of having a cesarean operation can be financially devastating.

Although the majority of American women do have health insurance that covers maternity care, only about 8 percent of these policies cover all maternity bills. The vast majority of health insurance policies require both deductibles and copayments. A deductible is a certain amount of money you must pay after the insurance coverage takes effect. A copayment is a percentage of the bill that you have to pay even after the deductible has been paid.

Insurance companies have been hit hard by the skyrocketing U.S. cesarean section rate. To cover their part of the additional hospital and doctor bills these companies have had to come up with an additional two thousand dollars or so for each cesarean section performed. Hence, the 935,000 cesarean operations performed in 1987 cost the insurance companies $1,870,000,000 more than if all these babies had been delivered normally. This estimate is very rough, but over a billion dollars is a lot of money! Thus, insurance companies are taking a very close look at the country's number one operation.

For example, the *Register* recently reported that Blue Shield, one of the nation's largest health insurance companies, is now checking on *every* cesarean section at all 225 hospitals in California.[6] If an insurance company concludes that a given cesarean section was unnecessary, it may refuse to pay for the surgery. As a precaution, you might want to check with your health insurance company before deciding to have an elective or routine repeat cesarean section.

Who Decides Whether or Not to Do a Cesarean?

To some people the obvious answer is that this decision is a medical one. Others would strongly disagree and claim that it's the woman's decision. These two opposing points of view aren't necessarily unreconcilable, since one involves the decision to perform surgery and the other the consent to do so. With a few rare exceptions, no operation can be performed without the written consent of the patient. For example, when doing a breast biopsy in an anesthetized woman, a doctor might conclude that a lump is malignant. However, he or she can't proceed with a mastectomy without obtaining prior written permission from the patient. For this reason a doctor must either agree that no major surgery will be performed at the time of a biopsy or must obtain the patient's written consent to proceed with more radical surgery at his or her discretion. The rule that the patient gives permission prior to surgery is true for any type of operation unless the individual is mentally incompetent and unable to give informed consent.*

From the above discussion one might assume that since a person must give written permission prior to undergoing surgery, the final decision regarding VBAC would be up to the mother. This assumption isn't necessarily true. Suppose a couple decides that they want a VBAC but their doctor only does repeat cesarean sections. The doctor cannot proceed with surgery without written permission, but to the best of my knowledge the woman cannot force the doctor to go along with VBAC. Hopefully this situation will not arise very often now that the American College of

---

*In obstetrics there is one very unusual exception to this rule. If a fetus appears to be in serious trouble, and the mother refuses to undergo a cesarean operation, the doctor can, in rare instances, obtain a court order to proceed with surgery against the mother's will. This situation is one of the only ones in modern times where an individual can be forced to undergo surgery against his or her will.

Obstetricians and Gynecologists has come out strongly in favor of VBAC. (See also chapter 9.)

If the doctor agrees to allow VBAC, then a decision has been made against elective cesarean section. But this decision does not guarantee a natural childbirth. At any time during the labor, the decision about whether or not to perform a cesarean section may again arise. Since you may be tired and under the influence of medications, sound decisions may be difficult to make. For this reason it would be a good idea to talk to your doctor prior to labor so that you can reach a mutually acceptable agreement about what to expect.

It is clearly wise to avoid any operation that is not necessary, but one's goal should never be to avoid surgery at any cost. At times, cesarean is actually the safest method of birth. Early in this book the history of cesarean was reviewed and it was shown that many women died due to complications of the operation. But it must be emphasized that today the chance of a woman dying during childbirth is extremely low, regardless of whether she delivers vaginally or by cesarean section. Many experts agree that some of the one million cesarean sections performed in this country every year are, to put it bluntly, unnecessary. But it must be remembered that some of these operations are absolutely necessary. A few years ago a colleague of mine cared for a woman who refused a cesarean operation in spite of fetal monitoring that indicated her baby was in serious trouble. I'm not the world's biggest advocate of electronic fetal monitoring, and unless viewed with some skepticism, these supposedly worrisome monitor findings can lead to needless cesarean operations. But in this case the fetal monitor results were simply horrendous. Unfortunately, the woman continued to refuse to be taken to the operating room and several hours later her baby died. The outcome was devastating for the couple and for the labor coach who had urged them not to consent to surgery. The lesson to be learned from this tragic story is that cesarean should not be viewed as an evil to be avoided at any cost. Striving to eliminate unnecessary surgery is an honorable goal, but we must never forget that, at times, the cesarean operation can be lifesaving.

CHAPTER 12

The Future of Birth

Birth has two meanings. One has to do with objective mechanical things like how a baby actually gets out of its mother's body. The other has to do with less tangible things like maternal instincts and mother-infant bonding. These subjective aspects of birth, the psychological and sociological consequences of the event, are so complex that entire books have been written on the subject. So, let's simplify our discussion and stick to the mechanical aspects of childbirth.

First, how does the mother's body know when the baby is ready to be born? What starts the process of labor? Nobody knows the answer! There are several current theories, most having to do with complex biochemical mechanisms, but no one knows for sure. Some scientists believe that the baby itself, perhaps by sending out some kind of hormone, initiates the process of labor in its mother's body. Hundreds of doctors around the world are trying to answer the question, because if they can, they might be able to reverse the process and come up with a miracle drug that will stop premature labor, the number one cause of infant mortality.

Let's put aside the question of what starts labor and get to the real issue at hand. What is birth? We can look at this from two points of view: the baby's and the mother's. The baby, who's been calmly floating in amniotic fluid for many months, must suddenly make several amazing transitions, all within the course of a few hours. Perhaps the most amazing will be the transition from existing completely underwater to living in an air-filled world.

In addition to breathing, the baby will suddenly have to take over a host of functions that the mother's body has been providing. The infant, who has been kept at a constant 98.6 degrees F in nature's perfect incubator, will suddenly have to regulate its own temperature. The constant flow of nutrients, the glucose and the predigested proteins, will suddenly be cut off and the newborn will have to take over its own digestive and metabolic functions. Much like a space shuttle in the tense moments as it clears its launch platform, a baby, once cut loose from the umbilical cord, is on its own.

Now let's look at birth from the mother's point of view. A little person, a miniature replica of the two parents, has slowly been developing deep within the mother's body. After about forty weeks of development the child is finally ready to come out. How is this little person going to get out? We're not talking about a creature the size of a marble or even a hen's egg. We're talking about a package that's twenty inches long and weighs seven or eight pounds! By some amazing process that even the most brilliant physicians can't fully understand, the baby will indeed pass from deep within your body to the outside world. The cervix will open, the uterus will contract, and the infant will negotiate the birth canal. It's happened a trillion times before. And, yes, it happened a trillion times before modern surgeons ever dreamed of the cesarean operation.

But let's not forget the other creatures with whom we

share this wonderful planet. What about the horses and cows and sheep and zebras? Birth seems to have worked rather well for them too. If their numbers dwindle it will not be because the process of birth has failed them. How many rabbits have been born in, say, the last thousand years? How many kittens? The list goes on and on. How many times has the process of birth been tested on this planet? Fifty trillion? A million zillion? The number is too large to even begin to contemplate.

Whether we believe in evolution, or divine creation, or some combination of the two, we must all agree that an amazing process exists. This process causes a fetus to pass from its mother's body and simultaneously prepares it to function as an independent entity. We call this miraculous process *birth*.

Is Natural Birth Doomed?

It may be, at least in developed countries. In the United States, for example, some people would argue that natural birth has already been virtually eliminated. To these people, natural birth means exactly what the name implies, "natural," as it would occur in nature, with no intervention or interference whatsoever. An example would be an unattended home birth where no medications or monitors are used. This method of childbirth, which served humankind well for millenniums, has indeed become rare in the United States. Interestingly, the entire process of changing natural birth to a medical procedure has taken, at most, a few generations. It is true that there are still a few holdouts who practice truly "natural" birth. These individuals generally fall into two groups: those who refuse modern high-tech obstetric care for religious reasons and those who reject such care on the grounds that it has little or no value.

But even if we pool all of the "natural" births achieved by members of these two groups together, and even if we include all of the "accidental natural births" (for example, women who give birth at home before they can get a ride to the hospital), the total incidence of truly "natural" births probably numbers only in the thousands. That figure pales by comparison against the 3 million to 4 million babies who are delivered by "conventional" means in American hospitals each year.

So it would appear that truly natural childbirth may be doomed in the United States. The real question becomes, "Is this a good thing or a bad thing?" The answer would depend on who you talk to. Most obstetricians think it's a wonderful thing! It's probably safe to say that most obstetricians consider those who totally reject modern obstetrical care to be lunatics. On the opposite side of the fence, many members of the childbirth reform movement believe that the elimination of natural birth was nothing less than an atrocity. As with so many other arguments, the true answer probably lies somewhere in between these two opposing points of view. Modern obstetrical techniques have undoubtedly saved many babies from death and disability. But some would ask, "At what cost?"

Is Normal Birth Doomed?

This question does not refer to "natural" birth. I'm not asking if home birth is doomed or if birth without fetal monitors is doomed. And I'm no longer talking about women who have had previous cesarean sections. As outrageous as the question may sound, I'm actually asking if the entire concept of normal vaginal birth will be eliminated. In other words, will cesarean section become the only way to have a baby?

I'll admit that this question sounds totally ridiculous, but before you dismiss the concept as an absurdity please read the following sentence. On May 9, 1985, the *New England Journal of Medicine* published a four-page article advocating that *all* women, even women with absolutely no medical indication for surgery, be offered the option of cesarean section.[1]

The premise of that article, written by Doctors Feldman and Freiman of New York, was that by surgically removing all infants at term, some babies would be spared the complications that occasionally arise during labor. They contended that perhaps one out of two hundred babies are in some way injured during labor and that these injuries could be eliminated by simply doing away with normal vaginal birth! The doctors did acknowledge that cesarean section was much riskier for the mother and that perhaps two to four times more mothers would die. But they claimed that the additional maternal deaths resulting from all these operations might be offset by the number of babies saved.

My first reaction to the article was that it was some kind of joke. I quickly searched through the rest of the journal hoping to find an explanation stating that the discussion on pages 1264 through 1267 was simply a satire on the rapidly rising United States cesarean rate. But there was no such explanation. I shared the article with several of my colleagues, both doctors and nurse-midwives. They all had the same reaction—it had to be some kind of joke. But it wasn't.

I spent the next weekend typing and retyping a fiery letter to the editor of the *New England Journal of Medicine*. Below is an excerpt from that letter:

> With the article "Prophylactic Cesarean Section at Term," Doctors Feldman and Freiman may have opened the door to the future of obstetrics. In the past few years there have already been an incredible number of changes in this field. We have seen the cesarean section rate *triple* in less than a decade. Feldman and Freiman conclude from their calculations that a shift toward *routine* cesarean section might "save a substantial number of potentially healthy infants at a *relatively low cost of excess maternal mortality*.." This con-

clusion is suspect for several reasons. Their assumption that the additional loss of mothers, who would die due to surgical complications, could be offset by fewer fetal losses is absurd. While the loss of a fetus near term is devastating, the needless death of a healthy young mother is inexcusable! Their assumption that iatrogenic prematurity could be reduced to zero by "adherence to protocols" is purely hypothetical.

Their conclusion that cost is not a major factor for those who currently undergo cesarean is also open to question. Estimates for the additional cost of each 1 percent increase in the cesarean section rate in the United States (thirty-five thousand additional operations) range from 63 *million* to 92 *million* dollars. Thus, even a 10 or 15 percent increase in the cesarean section rate would add a *billion* dollars a year to the health-care budget of a nation where 35 million people can't even afford basic health insurance.

But let us not dwell on technicalities. Let us assume for a moment that, through the miracle of modern technology, all maternal and fetal risks of cesarean section could be reduced to zero. Let us also assume that these operations could be performed at no additional cost, and that the network of operating rooms needed to perform an additional 3 million to 4 million operations each year could be quickly built and staffed. Allowing all of these incredible assumptions, and assuming that perhaps one out of three hundred infants would be saved from the supposed dangers of normal vaginal birth, let me ask one question: Does the natural physiologic process we call "birth" have no value?

The editor chose not to publish my letter. However, the *New England Journal of Medicine* did publish a letter from a doctor in Arizona. An excerpt follows:

I began reading "Prophylactic Cesarean Section at Term" with amusement, thinking that Drs. Feldman and Freiman were parodying some of the more interventionist obstetrical literature. Then, to my dismay, I discovered that they were serious.

I'd like to leave you with a parting thought. Although the vision of virtually all babies being delivered by cesarean section may seem totally ludicrous, please remember that the seeds of this vision have already been sewn in a major medical journal. Also remember that today in many American hospitals *one out of every three* babies is already delivered by the cesarean operation.

ADDENDUM

As this book goes to press I am completing the world's largest study on vaginal birth after cesarean section. This multicenter study began in 1984 and initially included nine California hospitals. During the first two years there were 1,776 trials of labor resulting in 1,304 vaginal births. Many of the results from these first two years are summarized in this book.

In January of 1986 two additional hospitals joined the collaborative project. Over the next three years there were 4,008 trials of labor resulting in 2,960 vaginal births at the eleven participating hospitals. During the entire five-year study period 5,784 patients opted for trial of labor and 4,264 (74 percent) delivered vaginally. There were no maternal deaths. Perinatal mortality was not significantly different from that of the general obstetrical population.

At these eleven hospitals, 4,264 women were able to successfully avoid repeat cesarean operations and all of the risks and complications associated with major surgery. These results strongly support the findings of approximately fifty other VBAC studies published over the past forty years. These studies have uniformly concluded that vaginal birth after cesarean section is both safe and likely to succeed.

APPENDIX A

Getting Help

Organizations That Help Women with Prior Cesareans

The rapidly rising United States cesarean section rate has caused a great deal of concern among advocates of natural childbirth. This concern has prompted the formation of several national consumer organizations. The Cesarean Prevention Movement Inc. (CPM) was founded in 1982 by Esther Zorn. CPM has more than sixty-five local chapters both in the United States and abroad. One of the principal goals of this organization is the promotion of vaginal birth after cesarean section. CPM is compiling consumer-based VBAC information nationwide and also publishes a quarterly newsletter called *The Clarion*. Birthworks, CPM's comprehensive childbirth preparation course, offers specific instruction for women with previous cesarean sections. Information about local chapters can be obtained from the national headquarters at the following address: Cesarean

Prevention Movement Inc., P.O. Box 152, Syracuse, New York 13210 (telephone 315/424–1942).

Cesareans/Support, Education and Concern (C/SEC) is another large consumer organization that was formed in response to U.S. skyrocketing cesarean section rates. For information write to C/SEC Inc., 22 Forest Road, Framingham, Massachusetts 01701 (telephone 617/877–8266).

The National Association of Parents and Professionals for Safe Alternatives in Childbirth (NAPSAC), founded by David and Lee Stewart, is based on the principle of freedom of choice in childbirth. For more information write to NAPSAC, P.O. Box 267, Marble Hill, Missouri 63764.

To the best of my knowledge these organizations are nonprofit and exist solely to further the cause of natural childbirth. Although the goals of all of these organizations are honorable, it should be noted that some of their recommendations have not been thoroughly evaluated by medical research. For example, some individuals have advocated VBAC at home and VBAC with prior classical cesarean sections. I caution you that essentially all physicians would agree that these are untested and perhaps dangerous options.

Getting More Information About VBAC

The references listed at the end of this book include dozens of medical studies on VBAC. Most of these reports can be found in any medical school library. There are more than one hundred medical schools in the United States and most people live within an hour's drive from one of them. If there is no medial school in your area, most large hospitals also have medical libraries. Medical librarians are generally very helpful to individuals seeking information from the medical literature.

A good source of information about cesarean section statistics is the Public Citizen Health Research Group. The group, which recently published a report entitled "Unnecessary Cesarean Sections: A Rapidly Growing National Epidemic," is now gathering cesarean section data from all over the country. They can be reached at 2000 P Street, N.W., Suite 700, Washington, D.C. 20036.

Childbirth educators are also good sources of information about birth after cesarean section. Childbirth educators can also be helpful in referring you to a doctor or nurse-midwife who has a special interest in normal birth after cesarean section. Nurses who work in the labor and delivery area of a hospital are another good source of information.

The two largest organizations of childbirth educators are the American Society of Psychoprophylaxsis in Obstetrics (ASPO/Lamaze) and the International Childbirth Education Association (ICEA). Each has chapters all over the United States and could probably refer you to a VBAC instructor in your area. Write to:

ASPO/Lamaze
1840 Wilson Boulevard, Suite 204
Arlington, Virginia 22201
Telephone (703) 524-7802

ICEA
P.O. Box 20048
Minneapolis, Minnesota 55420-0048
Telephone (612) 854-8660

American Academy of Husband-Coached Childbirth (AAHCC)
P.O. Box 5224
Sherman Oaks, California 91413
Telephone (213) 788-6662 (Bradley method)

Information about certified nurse-midwives can be obtained from:

The American College of Nurse-Midwifery (ACNM),
15 K Street, N.W., Suite 1120
Washington, D.C. 20005
Telephone (202) 347-5445

Midwives Alliance of North America (MANA)
30 South Main
Concord, New Hampshire 03301
Telephone (603) 225-9586

Consortium for Nurse-Midwifery, Inc. (CNMI)
1911 West 233rd Street
Torrance, California 90501
Telephone (213) 539-9801
(Information about nurse-midwifery in California)

Information about VBAC in Canada can be obtained from the following organizations:

VBAC of British Columbia
c/o Maternal Health Society
P.O. Box 46563, Station G
Vancouver, B.C. V6R 4G8, Canada

VBAC of Ontario
70 Ferncroft Drive
Scarborough, Ontario M1N 2X4, Canada

Cesarean Birth Association of Montreal
401 Boulevard St. Jean
Pointe Claire, Quebec H9R 3J3, Canada

APPENDIX B

ACOG Committee
Statements on VBAC

(NOTE: The American College of Obstetricians and Gynecologists (ACOG) is the world's largest organization of OB/GYN specialists. The following guidelines were issued by ACOG in 1988.)

Of the more than 3.7 million babies born each year in the United States, approximately 24 percent are delivered by cesarean birth, and one in three of these are repeat cesarean deliveries (1). Although for many years physicians in Western European countries have not regarded a previous low transverse uterine incision as a contraindication to subsequent labor and vaginal delivery, this practice is only now beginning to be followed in the United States.

In 1980, the National Institute of Child Health and Human Development Conference on Childbirth concluded that vaginal delivery after cesarean birth is an appropriate option (2). Current data show that a trial of labor was successful in 50 percent to 80 percent of patients who had low transverse uterine incisions from previous deliveries and who were selected candidates for vaginal birth in subsequent pregnancies. Moreover, a trial of labor was successful in this selected group in up to 70 percent of women for whom the indication for cesarean delivery was "failure to progress in labor." The data also indicate that maternal and perinatal mortality rates for subsequent attempted vaginal delivery are lower than those for repeat cesarean births (3–10). Although uterine rupture can occur, it is rarely catastrophic with modern obstetric care. The benefits of a successful vaginal delivery include elimination of operative and postoperative complications and shortened hospital stay.

It has been suggested in several reports that women who have had more than one prior cesarean delivery can be safely allowed a trial of labor (11, 12). The data reveal that the maternal and fetal risks for these women do not seem to be greater than those for women with only one previous cesarean delivery.

There are insufficient data to assess the safety or danger of labor for women with a previous low vertical incision. Likewise, the effects of labor on patients with more than one fetus, a breech presentation, or an estimated fetal weight of more than 4,000 g have not been substantiated.

Each hospital should develop its own protocol for management of patients who are encouraged to deliver vaginally after a previous cesarean birth. Suggested guidelines include the following:

1. The concept of routine repeat cesarean birth should be replaced by a specific indication for a subsequent abdominal delivery, and in the absence of a contraindication, a woman with one previous cesarean delivery with a low transverse incision should be counseled and encouraged to attempt labor in her current pregnancy.
2. A woman with two or more previous cesarean deliveries with low transverse incisions who wishes to attempt vaginal birth should not be discouraged from doing so in the absence of contraindications.
3. In circumstances in which specific data on risks are lacking, the question of whether to allow a trial of labor must be assessed on an individual basis.

4. A previous classical uterine incision is a contraindication to labor.

5. Professional and institutional resources must have the capacity to respond to acute intrapartum obstetric emergencies, such as performing cesarean delivery within thirty minutes from the time the decision is made until the surgical procedure is begun, as is standard for any obstetric patient in labor.

6. Normal activity should be encouraged during the latent phase of labor; there is no need for restriction to a labor bed before actual labor has begun.

7. A physician who is capable of evaluating labor and performing a cesarean delivery should be readily available.

Because of the potential risk of uterine rupture with the administration of oxytocin, some physicians choose not to use it to induce or augment labor for patients who have undergone a prior cesarean delivery (1). Recent reports indicate, however, that the use of oxytocin for augmentation of labor confers no greater risk upon patients undergoing a trial of labor after prior cesarean delivery with low transverse incision than upon the general population (13, 14).

Although controversy exists over the type of anesthesia that can be administered during labor for women with prior cesarean birth (2, 7), there is no evidence that epidural anesthesia is contraindicated in these patients (9, 10, 12).

REFERENCES

1. Placek, P. J., S. M. Taffel, and M. Moien. 1988. "1986 C-Sections Rise; VBACs Inch Upward." *Am. J. Public Health* 78(5):562–563.

2. U.S. Department of Health and Human Services; Public Health Service; National Institutes of Health. 1981. "Repeat Cesarean Birth." *Cesarean Childbirth*. NIH Publication No. 82-2067. U.S. Government Printing Office, Washington, D.C.

3. Boucher, M., M. P. Tahilramaney, G. S. Eglinton, et al. 1984. "Maternal Morbidity as Related to Trial of Labor After Previous Cesarean Delivery: A Quantitative Analysis." *J. Reprod. Med.* 29(1):12–16.

4. Phelan, J. P., G. S. Eglinton, J. M. Horenstein, et al. 1984. "Previous Cesarean Birth: Trial of Labor in Women with Macrosomic Infants." *J. Reprod. Med.* 29(1):36–40.

5. Martin, J. N., B. A. Harris, J. F. Huddleston, et al. 1983. "Vaginal Delivery Following Previous Cesarean Birth." *Am. J. Obstet. Gynecol.* 146(3):255–263.

6. Lavin, J. P., R. J. Stephens, M. Miodovnik, et al. 1982. "Vaginal Delivery in Patients with a Prior Cesarean Section." *Obstet. Gynecol.* 59(2):135–148.

7. Stovall, T. G., D. C. Shaver, S. K. Solomon, et al. 1987. "Trial of Labor in Previous Cesarean Section Patients, Excluding Classical Cesarean Sections." *Obstet. Gynecol.* 70(5):713–717.

8. Beall, M., G. S. Eglinton, S. L. Clark, et al. 1984. "Vaginal Delivery After Cesarean Section in Women with Unknown Types of Uterine Scar." *J. Reprod. Med.* 29(1):31–35.

9. Phelan, J. P., S. L. Clark, F. Diaz, et al. 1987. "Vaginal Birth After Cesarean." *Am. J. Obstet. Gynecol.* 157(6):1510–1515.

10. Flamm, B. L., O. W. Lim, C. Jones, et al. 1988. "Vaginal Birth After Cesarean Section: Results of a Multicenter Study." *Am. J. Obstet. Gynecol.* 158(5):1079–1084.

11. Porreco, R. P., and P. R. Meier. 1983. "Trial of Labor in Patients with Multiple Previous Cesarean Sections." *J. Reprod. Med.* 28(11):770–772.

12. Phelan, J. P., M. O. Ahn, F. Diaz, et al. 1988. "Twice a Cesarean, Always a Cesarean?" Abstract, 36th Annual Clinical Meeting. American College of Obstetricians and Gynecologists.

13. Horenstein, J. M., and J. P. Phelan. 1985. "Previous Cesarean Section: The Risks and Benefits of Oxytocin Usage in a Trial of Labor." *Am. J. Obstet. Gynecol.* 151(5): 564–569.

14. Flamm, B. L., J. R. Goings, N. J. Fuelberth, et al. 1987. "Oxytocin During Labor After Previous Cesarean Section: Results of a Multicenter Study." *Obstet. Gynecol.* 70(5): 709–712.

Summary of Medical Reports on VBAC in the United States

Although VBAC has become popular in the past decade, the concept of normal birth after cesarean section is certainly not a new one. In fact, very few medical topics have been subjected to such meticulous scientific scrutiny. What follows is a brief summary of some of the larger medical reports on VBAC. So many VBAC reports have been published over the past fifty years that it would be difficult to include all of them. Hence, smaller reports that include under one hundred women have been excluded.

Medical Reports on VBAC Published During the 1950s

In 1951, doctors at Lewis Hospital in Chicago reported on 106 women who had normal births after previous cesarean sections.[1] These births took place during 1931 to 1950.

Also in 1951, Dr. Robert Cosgrove reported on twenty years of experience with VBAC at the Margaret Hague Hospital in New Jersey.[2] Dr. Cosgrove's report included statistics on 221 VBAC mothers. In these two early reports a total of six babies were lost due to uterine rupture out of 327 VBACs (1.8 percent). But note that all six of these women had prior classical uterine incisions. Use of the classical type of uterine incision began to decline in the 1920s and this type of operation is rarely performed today.

Dr. Cosgrove noted that six mothers died due to complications of repeat cesarean operations. No mothers died in the group that delivered vaginally after previous cesarean section. It should be emphasized that the cesarean operation has become much less risky in recent years. Blood transfusions and powerful antibiotics that are available today could probably have saved some or all of the women described in Dr. Cosgrove's tragic report. Nevertheless, the fact that repeat cesarean section is a major operation with potential major complications should not be forgotten.

In 1956, a group of doctors in private practice in Chicago reported that during 1932 to 1955, 104 out of 107 women allowed to labor after previous cesarean section delivered vaginally.[3] Not a single uterine rupture occurred during their twenty-three years of allowing VBAC.

By the end of the 1950s, a sizable amount of data supporting the safety and efficacy of VBAC was already available. However, thirty years would pass before VBAC would become widely accepted in the United States.

Medical Reports on VBAC Published During the 1960s

In 1961, doctors at the Walter Reed Army Medical Center in Washington, D.C., reported on 202 women allowed to labor after previous cesarean section between 1953 and

1960. Of these women, 158 delivered vaginally. Interestingly, 22 of these women had more than one previous cesarean section. There were no serious complications among the mothers who opted for vaginal births, but one mother died due to hemorrhage after undergoing an elective repeat cesarean operation.[4]

In 1963, Doctor Douglas and his colleagues in New York reported on their experience with more than seven hundred VBACs during the prior thirty years.[5] In 1967, doctors at the Margaret Hague Hospital in New Jersey published a continuation of the work originally reported by Dr. Cosgrove in 1951. The new report covered the years 1948 through 1961 and included 1,486 VBACs.[6] Although this report was published decades ago, the doctors reached profound conclusions, some that are only now being appreciated.

Cesarean section is a major operative procedure. If performed unnecessarily in a particular instance, it assumes, and justly deserves, the same onus as that reserved for any type of unnecessary operation.

The facilities required for the proper conduct of labor in a patient with a history of delivery by cesarean section should be an integral part of every hospital with a qualified obstetric department.

Vaginal delivery following prior cesarean section in selected cases is certainly as safe—and probably safer—for mother and child than is elective repeat cesarean section.

By the end of the 1960s, doctors in the United States had already reported thousands of successful VBACs. Doctors in other countries had reported thousands more.

Medical Reports on VBAC Published During the 1970s

In 1978, doctors at the University of Texas reported that 313 out of 526 women allowed to labor after previous cesarean section delivered vaginally.[7] It was concluded that, "In general, the benefits of trial of labor included the decreased morbidity and reduced expenses in the 50 percent of patients who delivered vaginally." (Note that more recent studies indicate that about 75 percent of mothers who attempt VBAC will succeed.)

In 1979, doctors at the Albert Einstein College of Medicine in New York reported on labor in 145 women with prior cesarean sections.[8] Interestingly, 38 of these women had more than one prior cesarean section. Over a decade ago these doctors concluded that "There does not seem to be any rational or scientific basis for a 99 percent repeat cesarean rate in the United States and most well-equipped centers in the United States should abandon this practice."

Medical Reports on VBAC Published During the 1980s

In 1980, doctors at the University of Texas published an update of their original 1978 report.[9] The new report included a total of 1,192 trials of labor resulting in 746 successful VBACs. Not a single baby was lost due to the supposedly treacherous uterine rupture. The doctors concluded that "Once a section, always a section was appropriate for a previous time."

A report from doctors in Colorado in 1982 described 175 VBACs out of 207 women who tried for normal birth.[10] There were no maternal or perinatal deaths. The physicians concluded that "Trial of labor is not just an acceptable alternative to elective repeat cesarean delivery but is, indeed, the best medical practice."

In 1983, doctors in Mississippi and Alabama reported on the results of labor in 165 women with prior cesareans.[11] Of these women 101 (62 percent) delivered vaginally. None of the mothers or babies had any serious complications.

A report from the state of Washington published in 1984 noted that 69 percent of 242 women allowed to labor had successful VBACs.[12] One conclusion reached was that "The uniformity of the reports showing safe and successful results with trial of labor suggests that the persistence of elective repeat cesarean section is based on philosophical rather than scientific reasons."

Also in 1984, a report from the University of California indicated that VBAC was safe even if oxytocin was required to stimulate the labor and even if epidural analgesia was used.[13] Out of 230 women who attempted VBAC, 181 (79 percent) were able to avoid surgery. The doctors concluded that "Cesarean sections should be performed to protect the mother or the fetus. Elective repeat cesarean section frequently does not achieve either goal."

Recently, several reports about VBAC have come from the University of Southern California Medical Center.[14,15] In separate studies published in 1984, 1985, and 1987, a total of 2,104 women attempted VBAC and 1,705 (81 percent) succeeded. Note that since many of the patients at USC had their primary cesarean sections in other countries, it was not possible to document the type of uterine incision in the majority of cases. In spite of this fact, the majority of prior cesarean mothers at their medical center are allowed to deliver vaginally. After many years of research the doctors at USC concluded that "The benefits associated with a trial of labor in the patient with a prior cesarean birth far outweigh the risks. The policy of 'Once a cesarean section, always a cesarean section' should be abandoned."

A report from the University of Vermont published in 1985 revealed that 142 out of 216 women who attempted vaginal birth after cesarean succeeded in avoiding repeat operation.[16] There were no serious complications in any of these cases.

A very important medical report came out of the University of Texas in 1986.[17] Doctors studied 1,156 women who went through labor after a previous cesarean section. Of these women, 745 had vaginal births. It was found that the need for emergency cesarean section was no higher in the previous cesarean mothers than it was in any other laboring women. This study was important since many hospitals had not allowed VBAC on the grounds that VBAC mothers were supposedly at higher risk for requiring emergency surgery. The revised ACOG guidelines for VBAC now indicate that any hospital that is adequately equipped for childbirth is also adequately equipped for VBAC.

In 1987, physicians at the University of Tennessee College of Medicine reported that during a one-year period 216 out of 272 women who attempted VBAC succeeded.[18] Unlike most other reports on VBAC, this one included many women with prior vertical uterine incisions. The doctors concluded that "In summary, a trial of labor is a safe alternative for those patients with a single lower uterine segment *vertical* scar or transverse scar, as well as for patients with multiple uterine scars." Note that very few studies have included women with prior vertical uterine scars and hence it may be too soon to conclude that labor is safe with this type of scar. In any case, the vast majority of cesarean section scars are of the low transverse type, *not* the vertical type.

On rare occasions it is may not be possible to determine what type of scar you have on your uterus. For example, if your medical records have been destroyed in a fire, you may not be able to obtain a copy of your operative report. Since many of the patients at Baylor College of Medicine in Houston, Texas, are indigent and have inconsistent prenatal care, previous cesarean mothers often present in labor before old medical records can be obtained. In 1988, the doctors at Baylor reported on 300 women who attempted VBAC with an unknown type of uterine scar.[19] Sixty-two percent of these women had successful VBACs and the incidence of uterine scar rupture was not increased.

The Texas physicians concluded that "Allowing a trial of labor in a patient with an unknown uterine scar does not place the mother or fetus at greater risk than for a patient with a known low cervical transverse incision."

In 1988, a group of doctors from Tacoma, Washington, reported that 227 women had attempted VBAC and 167 (74 percent) had avoided repeat operation.[20] The doctors noted that even women who had an initial cesarean section for dystocia, or failure to progress in labor, had a 68 percent chance of a successful VBAC. The doctors concluded that "Unless there is well-documented evidence of cephalopelvic disproportion (abnormal pelvic bones), all patients with a history of dystocia should be considered for trial of labor. A successful outcome can be anticipated in approximately two-thirds of these women."

A similar 1988 study from Northwestern University Medical School in Chicago, Illinois, revealed that even women with previous cesarean sections for failure to progress or cephalopelvic disproportion were very likely to have successful VBACs if given a chance.[21] Specifically, the doctors at Northwestern concluded that "Patients with a prior cesarean section for arrest of labor are good candidates for a trial of labor and the cervical dilatation previously reached does not determine the likelihood of success."

In a multicenter study of nine hospitals in California during 1984 and 1985, 1,776 women attempted VBAC.[22] Of these women 1,314 (74 percent) had successful vaginal births. This statistic was true in spite of the fact that the majority of these women (649) had a first cesarean section because of failure to progress in labor. Of these women, 89 had a history of two or more prior cesarean sections. I was the director of this multicenter project and hence I can personally attest to the safety and efficacy of VBAC.

By the close of the 1980s, thousands upon thousands of successful VBACs had been documented in literally dozens of medical reports from all over the United States. In contrast, a comprehensive review of the medical literature failed to reveal even a single medical report that came out in favor of routine repeat cesarean section.

. . . .

APPENDIX D

. . . .

Summary of Medical Reports on VBAC from Around the World

For several years I've been collecting VBAC reports from all over the world. But please note that the following list is by no means all encompassing! In the summary that follows I have included only papers published in English or papers with an English abstract. Each year reports from all over the world continue to document the safety of VBAC.

VBAC Reports from Africa

In 1983, doctors at the University of Zambia published the results of labor in 319 women with prior cesarean sections.[1] Of these women, 201 (63 percent) delivered vaginally. There were no major complications and the doctors concluded that "Parturition in otherwise obstetrically normal patients seems to be safe, and the trial of labor approach is desirable as it results in a lower number of repeat cesarean operations."

A report from Johannesburg, South Africa, published in 1986, found VBAC to be safe even when oxytocin was needed to stimulate labor.[2] The South African doctors noted that "It should be remembered that the neonatal benefits of an increased cesarean section rate must be weighed against the costs of increased maternal mortality and morbidity."

In 1987, doctors at the University of Cape Town reported on 106 women who were allowed to labor after previous cesarean section at the Cecilia Makiwane Hospital in the rural Ciskei area of South Africa.[3] No maternal or fetal mortality occurred and it was concluded that with proper precautions labor after cesarean section was feasible even in rural Third World settings.

VBAC Reports from Austria

In 1986, doctors from the Medical University at Graz reported that of 261 women with prior cesarean sections, 166 had successful VBACs.[4]

VBAC Reports from Canada

Canada, like the United States, has been slow to accept VBAC. However, some Canadian doctors have taken an active interest in normal birth after cesarean section. For example, in 1982, doctors at McMaster University Health Sciences Center in Ontario reported on 92 women permitted to attempt vaginal delivery.[5] The Canadian doctors concluded that "There seems abundant evidence that Craigin's old dictum of 'once a cesarean section, always a cesarean section' initially applied to classical cesarean section, should be firmly abandoned."

VBAC Reports from Germany

A report from Germany in 1984 indicated that 57 percent of 565 women who had previously undergone a cesarean section were able to avoid cesarean section with their next pregnancy.[6] Interestingly, 71 percent of these women were given peridural analgesia (similar to epidural analgesia) during labor. The German physicians concluded that "Previous cesarean section is no indication for a repeat cesarean section."

In 1985, a medical report from Germany discussed VBAC and concluded that "Vaginal delivery of women with a history of cesarean section is not only perfectly feasible, but is connected with little risk provided mother and fetus are monitored with utmost care."[7]

VBAC Reports from Great Britain

In 1953, doctors at the Maternity Hospital at Leeds reported on 488 women allowed to labor after previous cesarean section.[8] Two years later doctors in Liverpool reported that 74 out of 83 women allowed to labor after prior cesarean section delivered vaginally.[9] In 1969, a report from Glasgow indicated that 242 out of 334 women with previous cesarean sections delivered vaginally in a single year at Queen Mother Hospital.[10] The doctors in Glasgow concluded that "After primary cesarean section, subsequent vaginal delivery is frequently possible and desirable."

In 1972, a very interesting report came out of Oxford in which 75 women with prior cesarean sections were given caudal (similar to epidural) analgesia during labor.[11] Of these women, 71 had successful VBACs. The doctors at Oxford concluded that "We consider that elective repeat cesarean section is meddlesome obstetrics unless there is a recurring indication." They also concluded that "Elective cesarean section without adequate justification usually subjects the patient to the dual insult of unnecessary general anesthesia and unnecessary surgery."

Another interesting report came out of Oxford University in 1984.[12] A group of doctors reviewed the results of induction of labor in 143 women with previous cesarean sections. Of these women, 108 (76 percent) went on to have a successful VBAC. All 143 women were given a medicine called prostaglandin to soften the cervix prior to induction of labor. This report is important since about 5 percent to 10 percent of women will go about two weeks past their due date. If this lateness happens to a woman with no previous cesarean section, most doctors recommend induction of labor (giving medicine to get the labor started). However, if a woman who has had a prior cesarean section goes significantly past her due date most American doctors recommend repeat cesarean section rather than induction of labor. This report indicates that it is safe to treat previous cesarean mothers who go past their due dates the same as any other woman. The English doctors concluded that "The method was simple, safe, and effective with 76 percent achieving a vaginal delivery and, even when the cervix was very unfavorable at the time of prostaglandin treatment, 68 percent achieved vaginal delivery. The procedure reduces the need for repeat cesarean section with its potential morbidity, without evidence of undue risk of lower segment scar rupture."

VBAC Reports from Hong Kong

Doctors at the Princess Margaret Hospital in Hong Kong reported that during 1980 to 1983, 666 women were allowed to labor after a previous cesarean section.[13] Of these women, 573 (86 percent) delivered vaginally. There were no serious complications with any of the mothers or babies. The physicians noted that even if the labor had to be induced, for example, in women who went significantly past their due date, VBAC was generally successful.

VBAC Reports from India

In 1987, doctors at Nehru Hospital in Chandigarh, India, reported that 590 women attempted VBAC and 452 (77 percent) had successful vaginal deliveries.[14] The overall perinatal mortality was actually higher in the group delivered by elective repeat cesarean section than in the VBAC group. The Indian doctors concluded that "The issue of 'once a section always a section' does not hold in present-day obstetrics."

Also in 1987, a report from the University Hospital in Varanasi, India, noted that 282 out of 468 women with previous cesarean sections delivered vaginally.[15] The doctors noted that "The cesarean section in modern obstetrics may be regarded as a double-edged sword."

VBAC Reports from Indonesia

A report from Jakarta published in 1983 noted that 93 out of 135 women with prior cesarean sections were able to give birth vaginally.[16] The Asian doctors concluded that "No significant increase in maternal and infant mortality was associated with women having vaginal delivery subsequent to cesarean birth as compared to those with repeat cesarean section."

VBAC Reports from Ireland

In 1963, doctors at the Rotunda Hospital in Dublin reported that out of 310 women allowed to labor after previous cesarean section 301 (97 percent) delivered vaginally.[17] Interestingly, 128 of these women had already had successful VBACs. Many women wonder if each successive VBAC will further stress the prior uterine scar. The Irish researchers found this fear to be unfounded. Many of their patients went on to have five or six vaginal births after an initial cesarean section. In fact, one woman actually had nine normal births after her initial cesarean section! A subsequent report from the same hospital published in 1965 included another 449 VBACs.[18]

In 1982, Dr. Dermot MacDonald reported on a twenty-year experience at the National Maternity Hospital in Dublin that included almost 2,500 VBACs.[19] In his discussion of why repeat cesarean section is so common in some parts of the world the Irish doctor raised some interesting points such as, "Perhaps patients are not given the choice, or the facts on which they could make a choice. Perhaps they have never been informed that there is an alternative to another section for them. The counseling must be based on factual truth and trust."

A study of 1,781 women attempting normal birth after cesarean section during 1979 to 1984 at Coombe Hospital in Dublin revealed that 1,618 (91 percent) delivered vaginally.[20] The Irish doctors concluded that "Labor may be safely allowed in women who have had a previous cesarean section, most of whom will deliver vaginally."

Considering the relatively small size of Ireland (1985 population of 3.5 million compared to the U.S. population of 239 million), it is intriguing that at least until the past few years the Irish have had more experience with VBAC than we have. Clearly, VBAC has been more popular in Europe than in the United States.

VBAC Reports from Israel

Doctors in Israel recently reported that it is safe to use epidural analgesia in women with previous cesarean sections. In a report published in 1984, 115 women with previous cesarean sections were given epidural analgesia for pain relief during labor.[21] Of these women, 102 (89 percent) had successful VBACs. The doctors concluded that "These results suggest that the use of epidural analgesia, using small doses of dilute bupivacaine solution, in the management of vaginal delivery after cesarean section is a safe approach." This report is significant since many American physicians still do not allow women with previous cesarean sections to have epidural analgesia during labor.

In 1987, doctors from Haifa, Israel, found that 215 out of 261 allowed to labor after previous cesarean section went on to have successful VBACs.[22] The Israeli doctors concluded that "The results of the present study compare favorably with other recent reports, indicating that more than two-thirds of properly selected patients allowed to labor will achieve a successful and safe vaginal delivery."

VBAC Reports from Italy

In 1985, doctors at the University of Milan in northern Italy reported that 101 women were allowed to labor after previous cesarean section and 77 had successful VBACs. No uterine ruptures occurred.[23]

VBAC Reports from Saudi Arabia

During 1983 to 1984, 1,446 women with previous cesarean operations attempted VBAC at the Maternity Hospital of

King Saud University in Saudi Arabia.[24] The perinatal mortality in these labors was actually lower than the overall rate for the hospital. The Arabian doctors concluded that "We have found that a trial of labor following previous cesarean section is often successful and should be used more often, thus reducing the risks associated with cesarean section."

VBAC Reports from South America

A report presented at the 1984 Chilean Society of Obstetrics and Gynecology discussed 227 successful VBACs.[25] The doctors discussed the issue of whether or not forceps should be used to shorten the pushing stage of labor in women with previous cesarean sections. They concluded that forceps had no benefits for VBAC mothers.

VBAC Reports from Spain

In 1988, doctors at the Hospital Nacional Valdecilla in Santander, Spain, reported that 202 out of 339 women with previous cesarean sections delivered vaginally.[26] No scar ruptures occurred. These results were from the first few years of a new VBAC program and the physicians felt that their VBAC success rate would improve as they became more comfortable with allowing labor after cesarean section. Specifically, the doctors concluded that "We think that the most interesting aspect of our results is that they probably represent the lower limit of what can be achieved safely with minimal technical means. Thus considered, they are a solid basis on which to improve.

VBAC Reports from Sweden

In 1980, doctors from the University Hospital at Lund published a report that focused on the use of epidural analgesia in women with prior cesarean sections.[27] Of the 119 women who attempted normal birth, 105 (88 percent) were able to avoid repeat cesarean section. The researchers concluded that it was reasonable to use epidural anesthesia in mothers with prior cesarean sections.

In 1989, doctors at the Central Hospital in Bords, Sweden, reported that 92 percent of 1,008 women attempting labor after previous cesarean section had successful VBACs.[28] The Swedish physicians concluded that "In summary, the risk of uterine rupture in patients who have previously undergone cesarean section but are allowed a trial of labor is low and not associated with serious complications. Vaginal delivery is therefore considered the safest route of delivery in these patients."

VBAC Reports from the West Indies

In 1973, doctors at the University Hospital of the West Indies at Kingston, Jamaica, reported that 171 out of 243 women (70 percent) allowed to labor after previous cesarean section delivered vaginally.[29] The doctors concluded that "In light of this experience, we must question the advisability of routine elective repeat cesarean section particularly when these patients are subjected to general anesthesia, blood transfusion, and increased postoperative mortality and morbidity, including wound infection, pulmonary and urinary infection, phlebitis and embolus, as well as an increase in hospital stay."

VBAC Reports from Yugoslavia

A report published in Serbo-Croatian (but fortunately abstracted in English!) reveals that of 452 women with previous cesarean section, 283 went on to deliver vaginally.[30]

Conclusion

This appendix has summarized the results of thirty medical reports from countries all over the world. These reports document thousands upon thousands of successful VBACs. In contrast, I was unable to find even a single medical report published anywhere in the world that came out in favor of routine repeat cesarean section.

When combined with the results of the twenty-two American VBAC reports summarized in appendix C, only one logical conclusion can be reached: Routine repeat cesarean section represents unnecessary major surgery. If all eligible women were allowed to deliver vaginally after previous cesarean section, more than 200,000 cesarean operations could be avoided in the United States each and every year.

....
NOTES
....

CHAPTER 1

1. U.S. Department of Health and Human Services, National Center for Health Statistics. 1986. "Utilization of Short-Stay Hospitals: Annual Summary for the United States." Data from the National Hospital Discharge Survey.
2. Steinbrook, R. August 21, 1988. "Runaway C-Section Rates Reflect Crisis." *Los Angeles Times.* p. 3.
3. U.S. Department of Health and Human Services. 1981. "Cesarean Childbirth." National Institutes of Health publication number 82-2076.
4. Winkler, J. D., D. E. Kanouse, L. Brodsley, and R. H. Brook. 1986. "Popular Press Coverage of Eight National Institutes of Health Consensus Development Topics." *J. Am. Med. Assoc.* 255:1323–1327.
5. Cosgrove, R. A. 1951. "Management of Pregnancy and Delivery Following Cesarean Section." *J. Am. Med. Assoc.* 145:884–888.
6. American College of Obstetrics and Gynecology. October 1988. "Guidelines for VBAC," second revision.

CHAPTER 2

1. Pritchard, J. A., and P. C. MacDonald. 1980. *Williams' Obstetrics*, 16th ed. ACC/Prentice-Hall, New York, pp. 1100–1101.
2. Speert, H. 1980. *Obstetrics and Gynecology in America: A History*. Waverly Press, Inc., Baltimore, p. 151.
3. Meigs, C. D. 1849. *Obstetrics: The Science and Art*. Lea and Blanchard Co., Philadelphia, p. 508.
4. Kerr, J. M. M. 1926. "The Technique of Cesarean Section with Special Reference to the Lower Uterine Segment Incision. *Am. J. Obstet. Gynecol.* 12:729.
5. Pritchard, J. A., and P. C. MacDonald. 1980. *Williams' Obstetrics*, 16th ed. ACC/Prentice-Hall, New York, pp. 1100–1101.
6. Harris, R. P. 1879. "A Study and Analysis of One Hundred Cesarean Operations Performed in the United States, During the Present Century, and Prior to the Year 1878." *Am. J. Med. Sci.* 77:43–65.
7. Paverstein, C. J. 1980. "Indications for Cesarean Delivery." *Clinical Obstetrics*. John Wiley & Sons, New York, p. 886.
8. Klein, L. 1984. "Cesarean Birth and Trial of Labor." *Female Patient* 9:106–117.
9. Cragin, E. B. 1916. "Conservatism in Obstetrics." *New York Med. J.* 104:1–3.

CHAPTER 3

1. U.S. Department of Health and Human Services. 1981. "Cesarean Childbirth." National Institutes of Health publication number 82-2076.
2. *Register*. July 30, 1985. "A Survey of Orange County Maternity Services." Orange County, California.

3. Public Citizen Health Research Group. 1989. "Unnecessary Cesarean Sections: How to Cure a National Epidemic." Washington, D.C.

4. Boulware, T. M., C. D. Howe, and S. T. Simpson. 1954. "A Discussion of Postpartum Sterilization." *Am. J. Obstet. Gynecol.* 68:1124–1128.

5. Kitchen, D., and R. S. Ledward. 1978. "Hazards of Multiple Cesarean Sections." *Practitioner* 220:786–788.

CHAPTER 4

1. Phelan, J. P., S. L. Clark, F. Diaz, and R. H. Paul. 1987. "Vaginal Birth After Cesarean Section." *Am. J. Obstet. Gynecol.* 157:1510–1515.

2. Flamm B. L., O. W. Lim, C. Jones, D. Fallon, L. A. Newman, and J. K. Mantis. 1988. "Vaginal Birth After Cesarean Section: Results of a Multicenter Study." *Am. J. Obstet. Gynecol.* 158:1079–1084.

3. Molloy, B. G., O. Sheil, and M. N. Duignan. 1987. "Delivery after Cesarean Section: Review of 2,176 Consecutive Cases." *Brit. Med. J.* 294:1645–1647.

4. Paul, R. H., J. P. Phelan, and S. Yeh. 1985. "Trial of Labor in the Patient with a Prior Cesarean Birth." *Am. J. Obstet. Gynecol.* 151:297–303.

CHAPTER 5

1. Evrard, J. R., and E. M. Gold. 1977. "Cesarean Section and Maternal Mortality in Rhode Island." *Obstet. Gynecol.* 50:594.

2. Klein, L. 1984. "Cesarean Birth and Trial of Labor." *Female Patient* 9:106–117.

3. U.S. Department of Health and Human Services. 1981. "Cesarean Childbirth." National Institutes of Health publication number 82-2076.

4. Endler, G. C., F. G. Mariona, R. J. Sokol, and L. B. Stevenson. 1988. "Anesthesia-related Maternal Mortality in Michigan, 1972–1984.

5. *Clinical Obstetrics.* 1987. Wiley, New York, pp. 887–888. And also "Pauerstein, Carl J. "Cesarean Delivery: Perioperative Complications." *Am. J. Obstet. Gynecol.* 159:187–193.

6. Gibbs, R. S. 1985. "Infection after Cesarean Section." *Clin. Obstet. Gynecol.* 4:697–710.

7. Pritchard, J. A., and P. C. MacDonald. 1980. *Williams' Obstetrics,* 16th ed. ACC/Prentice-Hall, New York, p. 235.

8. Eisenkop, S. M., R. Richman, L. D. Platt, and R. H. Paul. 1982. "Urinary Tract Injury During Cesarean Section." *Obstet. Gynecol.* 60:591–596.

9. Schaefer, G, and E. A. Graber. 1981. *Complications in Obstetrics and Gynecologic Surgery.* Harper & Row, New York, p. 36.

10. Queenan, J. T. 1988. "Cesarean Section." *Postgraduate Obstet. Gynecol.* 8:1–5.

11. Kistner, R. W., A. T. Hertig, and D. E. Reid. 1952. "Simultaneously Occurring Placenta Previa and Placenta Accreta." *Surg. Gynecol. Obstet.* 94:141–151.

12. Clark, S. L., P. P. Koonings, and J. P. Phelan. 1985. "Placenta Previa/Accreta and Prior Cesarean Section." *Obstet. Gynecol.* 66:89–92.

13. Affonso, D. D. 1981. *Impact of Cesarean Childbirth.* F. A. Davis Co., Philadelphia.

14. Flamm, B. L., et al. 1984. "Vaginal Birth after Previous Cesarean Section Allowing Oxytocin Augmentation and Epidural Anesthesia. *Am. J. Obstet. Gynecol.* 148:759–765.

15. Chervenak, F. A., et al. 1986. "Current Perspectives on Iatrogenic Neonatal Respiratory Distress Syndrome." *J. Reprod. Med.* 31:53–57.

16. Heritage, C. K., and M. D. Cunningham. 1985. "Association of Elective Repeat Cesarean Delivery and Persistent Pulmonary Hypertension of the Newborn." *Am. J. Obstet. Gynecol.* 152:627–629.

17. Schreiner, R. L., et al. 1982. "Respiratory Distress Following Elective Repeat Cesarean Section." *Am. J. Obstet. Gynecol.* 143:689–692.

18. Bowers, S. K., et al. 1982. "Prevention of Iatrogenic Neonatal Respiratory Distress Syndrome: Elective Repeat Cesarean Section and Spontaneous Labor." *Am. J. Obstet. Gynecol.* 143:186–189.

19. Zdeb, M. S., G. D. Therriault, and V. M. Logrillo. 1984. "Frequency, Spacing, and Outcome of Pregnancies Subsequent to Primary Cesarean Childbirth." *Am. J. Obstet. Gynecol.* 150:205–212.

20. Lee, B. T. 1985. "Cesarean Section and Future Childbearing." *Am. J. Obstet. Gynecol.* 152:363.

21. Hemminki, E. 1986. "Effects of Cesarean Section on Fertility and Abortions." *J. Reprod. Med.* 31:620–624.

22. LaSala, A. P., and A. S. Berkeley. 1987. "Primary Cesarean Section and Subsequent Infertility." *Am. J. Obstet. Gynecol.* 157:379–383.

CHAPTER 6

1. Shy, K. K., J. P. LoGerfo, and L. E. Karp. 1981. "Evaluation of Elective Repeat Cesarean Section as a Standard of Care: An Application of Decision Analysis." *Am. J. Obstet. Gynecol.* 139:123–129.

2. Silver, R. K., and J. Minogue. 1987. "When Does a Statistical Fact Become an Ethical Imperative?" *Am. J. Obstet. Gynecol.* 157:229–233.

3. American College of Obstetrics and Gynecology Guidelines for VBAC. January 1982. Initial Committee Statement.

4. American College of Obstetrics and Gynecology Guidelines for VBAC. November 1984. First revision.

5. American College of Obstetrics and Gynecology Guidelines for VBAC. October 1988. Second revision.

6. ICEA Position Statement: Cesarean Birth. 1980. *ICEA News* 19:3.
7. ICEA Review: Vaginal Birth after Cesarean Section. 1987. *Int. J Childbirth Education* 3:21–27.
8. ASPO/Lamaze, National Headquarters, 1840 Wilson Blvd., Suite 204, Arlington, VA 22201.
9. Frigoletto, F. D., G. A. Little, et al. 1988. *Guidelines for Perinatal Care*, 2nd ed. American Academy of Pediatrics, Elk Grove, IL.
10. U.S. Department of Health and Human Services. 1981. "Cesarean Childbirth." National Institutes of Health publication number 82-2076.
11. Notzon, F. C., P. J. Placek, and S. M. Taffel. 1987. "Comparison of National Cesarean Section Rates." *New Eng. J. Med.* 316:386–389.
12. Molloy, B. G., O. Sheil, and M. N. Duignan. 1987. "Delivery After Caesarean Section: Review of 2176 Consecutive Cases." *Brit. Med. J.* 294:1645–1647.
13. Meehan, F. P. 1988. "Delivery Following Prior Cesarean Section: An Obstetrician's Dilemma?" *Obstet. Gynecol. Survey* 43:582–589.
14. Canadian National Consensus Conference on Aspects of Cesarean Birth. "Indications for Cesarean Section." *Canadian Medical Association Journal* 134:1348–1352.
15. Austin, S. 1986. "Childbirth Classes for Couples Desiring VBAC." *Maternal Child Nursing* 11:250–255.
16. Placek, P. J., and S. M. Taffel. 1988. "Vaginal Birth After Cesarean (VBAC) in the 1980s." *Am. J. Public Health* 78:512–515.
17. Lavin, J. P., R. J. Stephens, M. Miodovnik, and T. P. Barden. 1982. "Vaginal Delivery in Patients with a Prior Cesarean Section." *Am. J. Obstet. Gynecol.* 59:135–148.

CHAPTER 7

1. Flamm B. L., et al. "Vaginal Birth After Cesarean Section: Results of a Multicenter Study. *Am. J. Obstet. Gynecol.* 158:1079–1084.

2. Flamm, B. L., et al. 1984. "Vaginal Birth After Previous Cesarean Section Allowing Oxytocin Augmentation and Epidural Anesthesia." *Am. J. Obstet. Gynecol.* 148:759–765.

3. Miller, J. M., et. al. "Estimated Fetal Weight." *J. Clinical Ultrasound* 16:95–97.

4. Phelan, J. P., et al. 1984. Trial of Labor in Women with Macrosomic Infants. *J. Reprod. Med.* 29:36–40.

5. Flamm, B. L., and J. Goings. 1989. "Vaginal Birth after Cesarean Section—Is Suspected Fetal Macrosomia a Contradiction?" *Obstetrics and Gynecology.* 74:694–697.

6. Benedetti, T. J., and S. G. Gabbe. 1978. "Shoulder Dystocia: Complication of Fetal Macrosomia." *Obstet. Gynecol.* 52:526–529.

7. National Center for Health Statistics. 1985. Advance Report of Final Natality Statistics, 1983. 34:6.

8. University of Washington herpes paper.

9. "Perinatal Herpes Simplex Infections." *ACOG HSV Bulletin 1988.*

10. Finley, B. E., and C. E. Gibbs. 1986. "Emergent Cesarean Delivery in Patients Undergoing a Trial of Labor with a Transverse Lower-Segment Scar." *Am. J. Obstet. Gynecol.* 155:936–939.

11. Paul, R. H., J. P. Phelan, and S. Yeh. 1985. Trial of Labor in the Patient with a Prior Cesarean Birth. *Am. J. Obstet. Gynecol.* 151:297–303.

12. Ibid., note 11.

13. Ibid., note 1.

CHAPTER 8

1. Finley, B. E., and C. E. Gibbs. 1986. "Emergent Cesarean Delivery in Patients Undergoing a Trial of Labor with a Transverse Lower-Segment Scar." *Am. J. Obstet. Gynecol.* 155:936–939.
2. Pritchard J. A., and P. C. Macdonald. 1980. *Williams' Obstetrics,* 16th ed. ACC/Prentice-Hall, New York, p. 410.
3. Crawford, J. S. 1972. "Maternal Mortality Associated with Anesthesia." *Lancet* 2:918.
4. Cameron, J. L., W. H. Mitchell, and G. D. Ziudema. 1973. "Aspiration Pneumonia: Clinical Outcome Following Documented Aspiration." *Arch. Surg.* 106:49.
5. Flamm, B. L. 1985. "Vaginal Birth After Cesarean Section: Controversies Old and New." *Clin. Obstet. Gynecol.* 28:735–745.
6. Case, B., R. Corcoran, and N. Jeffcoate. 1971. "Cesarean Section and Its Place in Modern Obstetric Practice." *J. Obstet. Gynecol. Br. Commonw.* 78:203–209.
7. Dhall, K., S. C. Mittal, V. Grover, and G. I. Dhall. 1987. "Childbirth Following Primary Cesarean Section: Evaluation of a Scoring System." *Int. J. Gynecol. Obstet.* 25:199–205.
8. Allahbadia, N. K. 1963. "Vaginal Delivery Following Cesarean Section." *Am. J. Obstet. Gynecol.* 85:241–249.
9. Placek, P. J., and S. M. Taffel. 1988. "Vaginal Birth After Cesarean (VBAC) in the 1980s." *Am. J. Public Health* 78:512–515.

CHAPTER 9

1. Flamm. B. L., J. R. Goings, N. J. Fuelberth, E. Fischermann, C. Jones, and E. Hersh. 1987. "Oxytocin During Labor After Previous Cesarean Section: Results of a Multicenter Study." *Obstet. Gynecol.* 70:709–712.

2. Sokol, R. J., M. G. Rosen, S. F. Bottoms, and L. Chik. 1981. "Risks Preceding Increased Primary Cesarean Birth Rates." *Obstet. Gynecol.* 59:340–346.

3. Pritchard, J. A., and P. C. MacDonald. 1980. *Williams' Obstetrics,* 16th ed. ACC/Prentice-Hall, New York, p. 787.

4. Lavin, J. P., R. J. Stephens, M. Miodovnik, and T. P. Barden. 1982. "Vaginal Delivery in Patients with a Prior Cesarean Section." *Am. J. Obstet. Gynecol.* 59:135–148.

5. Flamm, B. L. 1985. "Vaginal Birth After Cesarean Section: Controversies Old and New." *Clin. Obstet. Gynecol.* 28:735–745.

6. Horenstein, J. M., G. S. Eglinton, P. M. Tahilramaney, M. Boucher, and J. P. Phelan. 1984. "Oxytocin Use During Trial of Labor in Patients with Previous Cesarean Section." *J. Reprod. Med.* 29:26–30.

7. Finley, B. E., and C. E. Gibbs. 1986. "Emergent Cesarean Delivery in Patients Undergoing a Trial of Labor with a Transverse Lower-Segment Scar." *Am. J. Obstet. Gynecol.* 155:936–939.

8. Paul R. H., J. P. Phelan, and S. Yeh. 1985. "Trial of Labor in the Patient with a Prior Cesarean Birth." *Am. J. Obstet. Gynecol.* 151:297–303.

9. Shiono, P. H., J. G. Fielden, D. McNellis, G. G. Rhoads, and W. H. Pearse. 1987. "Recents Trends in Cesarean Birth and Trial of Labor Rates in the United States." *J. Am. Med. Assoc.* 257:494–497.

10. Phelan, J. P., S. L. Clark, R. P. Porreco, and J. P. VanDorsten. 1988. "Finding Alternatives to Cesarean Section." *Contemp. Obstet. Gynecol.* 1:191–210.

11. Tahilramaney, M. P., M. Boucher, G. S. Eglinton, M. Beal, and J. P. Phelan. 1984. "Previous Cesarean Section and Trial of Labor." *J. Reprod. Med.* 29:1721.

12. Paul, R. H., J. P. Phelan, and S. Yeh. 1985. "Trial of Labor in the Patient with a Prior Cesarean Birth." *Am. J. Obstet. Gynecol.* 151:297–303.

13. Allahbadia, N. K. 1963. "Vaginal Delivery Following Cesarean Section." *Am. J. Obstet. Gynecol.* 85:241–249.

14. Brady, K., and J. A. Read. 1988. "Vaginal Delivery of Twins After Previous Cesarean Section. *New Eng. J. Med.* 319:188–119.

15. Gilbert, L., N. Saunders, and F. Sharp. "The Management of Multiple Pregnancy in Women with a Lower-Segment Cesarean Scar." *British J. Obstet. Gynecol.* 95: 1312–1316.

16. Shiono, P. H., D. McNellis, and G. G. Rhoads. 1987. "Reasons for the Rising Cesarean Delivery Rates: 1978–1984." *Obstet. Gynecol.* 69:696–700.

17. Savona-Ventura, C. 1986. "The Role of External Cephalic Version in Modern Obstetrics." *Obstet. Gynecol. Survey* 41:393–400.

18. McGarry, J. A. 1969. "The Management of Patients Previously Delivered by Ceasarean Section." *J. Obstet. Gynecol. Brit. Commonw.* 76:137–143.

19. Dyson, D. C., J. E. Ferguson, and P. Hensleigh. 1986. "Antepartum External Cephalic Version Under Tocolysis." *Obstet. Gynecol.* 67:63–68.

20. Westgren, M. H., H. Edvall, L. Nordstrom, and E. Svalenius. 1985. "Spontaneous Cephalic Version of Breech Presentation in the Last Trimester." *British J. Obstet. Gynecol.* 92:19–22.

21. Phelan, J. P., M. O. Ahn, F. Diaz, H. S. Brar, and H. Rodriguez. May 1988. "Twice a Cesarean, Always a Cesarean?" Presented at the annual meeting of ACOG.

22. Duff, P., R. W. Huff, and R. S. Gibbs. 1984. "Management of Premature Rupture of Membranes and Unfavorable Cervix in Term Pregnancy." *Obstet. Gynecol.* 63:697–701.

23. Kappy, K. A., C. L. Cetrulo, R. A. Knuppel, C. J. Ingardia, et al. 1982. "Premature Rupture of Membranes at Term: Comparison of Induced and Spontaneous Labors." *J. Reprod. Med.* 27:29–33.

24. Beall, M., G. S. Eglinton, S. L. Clark, and J. P. Phelan. 1984. "Vaginal Delivery After Cesarean Section in Women with Unknown Types of Uterine Scar." *J. Reprod.* 29:31–35.

25. "Vital and Health Statistics: Detailed Diagnoses and Procedures." United States 1986. DHHS publication number (PHS) 88-1756.
26. Dewherst, C. 1957. "The Ruptured Caesarean Section Scar." *J. Obstet. Gynecol. Br. Emp.* 64:113–117.
27. Schwartz, S. I., et al. 1984. *Principles of Surgery,* 4th ed. McGraw-Hill, New York, p. 301.

CHAPTER 10

1. Laufer, A., V. Hodenius, L. Friedman, N. Duncan, C. M. Guy, S. MacPherson, and N. Barrows. 1987. VBAC: "Nurse-Midwifery Management." *J. Nurse-Midwifery* 32:41–47.
2. Wetz, R. W., and D. C. Wertz. 1977. *Lying-in: A History of Childbirth in America.* The Free Press/Macmillan Publishing Co., New York, p. 133.
3. Advance report of final natality statistics, 1983. National Center for Health Statistics. 1985, p. 6.
4. Ibid. note 1.
5. Berman, S., and V. Berman. 1986. *The Birth Center: An Approach to the Birth Experience.* Prentice Hall Press, New York.
6. American College of Obstetrics and Gynecology. "Guidelines for VBAC." October 1988. Second Revision.

CHAPTER 11

1. Evans, M. I., D. A. Richardson, J. S. Sholl, and B. A. Johnson. 1984. "Cesarean Section—Assessment of the Convenience Factor." *J. Reprod. Med.* 29:670–676.
2. Fraser, W., R. H. Usher, F. H. Mclean, et al. 1987. "Temporal Variation in Rates of Cesarean Section for Dystocia—Does Convenience Play a Role?" *Am. J. Obstet. Gynecol.* 156:300–304.
3. Health United States: 1987. The 12th annual report on the

health status of the nation submitted by the Secretary of Health to the President and Congress of the United States. 1988. DHHS publication number PHS 88-1232.

4. Gold, R. B., A. M. Kenney, and S. Singh. 1987. *Financing Maternity Care in the United States*. The Alan Guttmacher Institute. ISBN 0-939253-06-2.

5. Flamm, B. L., et al. 1984. "Vaginal Birth after Previous Cesarean Section Allowing Oxytocin Augmentation and Epidural Anesthesia." *Am. J. Obstet. Gynecol.* 148:759–765.

6. "Most Repeat Cesareans Unnecessary, Dangerous, Experts Say." The *Register*. June 20, 1988. Orange County, California, p. B3.

CHAPTER 12

1. Feldman, G. B., and J. A. Freiman. 1985. Prophylactic cesarean section at term. *New Eng. J. Med.* 312:1264–1267.

APPENDIX C

1. Schmitz, H., and C. Gajewski. 1951. "Vaginal Delivery Following Cesarean Section." *Am. J. Obstet. Gynecol.* 61:1232–1235.

2. Cosgrove, R. A. 1951. "Management of Pregnancy and Delivery Following Cesarean Section." *J. Am. Med. Assoc.* 145(12):884–888.

3. Lawler, P., M. Bulfin, F. Lawler, et al. 1956. "A Review of Vaginal Delivery Following Cesarean Section from Private Practice." *Am. J. Obstet. Gynecol.* 72:252–258.

4. Riva, H. L., and J. C. Teich. 1961. "Vaginal Delivery After Cesarean Section." *Am. J. Obstet. Gynecol.* 81(3): 501–510.

5. Douglas, R., S. Birnbaum, and F. MacDonald. 1963. "Pregnancy and Labor Following Cesarean Section." *Am. J. Obstet. Gynecol.* 86:961–968.

6. Donnelly, J., and K. Franzoni. 1967. "Vaginal Delivery Following Cesarean Section." *Obstet. Gynecol.* 29:871–879.

7. Merrill, B. S., and C. E. Gibbs. 1978. "Planned Vaginal Delivery Following Cesarean Section." *Obstet. Gynecol.* 52:50–52.

8. Saldana, L., H. Schulman, and L. Reuss. 1979. "Management of Pregnancy After Cesarean Section." *Am. J. Obstet. Gynecol.* 135:555–561.

9. Gibbs, C. E. 1980. "Planned Vaginal Delivery Following Cesarean Section." *Clinical Obstet. Gynecol.* 23(2): 508–515.

10. Meier, P. R., and R. P. Porreco. 1982. "Trial of Labor Following Cesarean Section: A Two-Year Experience. *Am. J. Obstet. Gynecol.* 144:671–678.

11. Martin, J. N., B. A. Harris, J. F. Huddleston, J. C. Morrison, M. G. Propst, W. L. Wiser, H. W. Perlis, and J. T. Davidson. 1983. "Vaginal Delivery Following Previous Cesarean Birth." *Am. J. Obstet. Gynecol.* 146:255–262.

12. Graham, R. A. 1984. "Trial Labor Following Previous Cesarean Section." *Am. J. Obstet. Gynecol.* 149:35–45.

13. Flamm, B. L., C. Dunnett, E. Fischermann, and E. J. Quilligan. 1984. "Vaginal Birth After Previous Cesarean Section Allowing Oxytocin Augmentation and Epidural Anesthesia." *Am. J. Obstet. Gynecol.* 148:759–765.

14. Paul, R. H., J. P. Phelan, and S. Yeh. 1985. "Trial of Labor in the Patient with Prior Cesarean Birth." *Am. J. Obstet. Gynecol.* 151:297–303.

15. Phelan, J. P., S. L. Clark, F. Diaz, and R. H. Paul. 1987. "Vaginal Birth After Cesarean Section." *Am. J. Obstet. Gynecol.* 157:1510–1515.

16. Jarrell, M. A., G. Ashmead, and L. G. Mann. 1985. "Vaginal Delivery After Cesarean Section: A Five-Year Study. *Obstet. Gynecol.* 63:628–632.

17. Finley, B. E., and C. E. Gibbs. 1986." Emergent Cesarean Delivery in Patients Undergoing a Trial of Labor, with a Transverse Lower-Segment Scar." *Am. J. Obstet. Gynecol.* 55:936–939.

18. Stoval, T. G., D. C. Shaver, S. K. Solomon, and G. D.

Anderson. 1987. "Trial of Labor in Previous Cesarean Section Patients, Excluding Classical Cesarean Sections." *Obstet. Gynecol.* 70:713–717.

19. Pruett, K. M., B. Kirshon, and D. B. Cotton. 1988. "Unknown Uterine Scar and Trial of Labor." *Am. J. Obstet. Gynecol.* 159:807–810.

20. Duff, P., K. Southmayd, and J. A. Read. 1988. "Outcome of Trial of Labor in Patients with a Single Previous Low Transverse Cesarean Section for Dystocia." *Obstet. Gynecol.* 71:380–384.

21. Ollendorff, D. A., J. M. Goldberg, J. P. Minogue, and M. L. Socol. 1988. "Vaginal Birth After Cesarean Section for Arrest of Labor." *Am. J. Obstet. Gynecol.* 159:636–639.

22. Flamm, B. L., O. W. Lim, C. Jones, D. Fallon, L. A. Newman, and J. K. Mantis. 1988. "Vaginal Birth After Cesarean Section: Results of a Multicenter Study." *Am. J. Obstet. Gynecol.* 158:1079–1084.

APPENDIX D

1. Wadhawan, S., and J. N. Narone. 1983. "Outcome of Labor Following Previous Cesarean Section." *Int. J. Gynecol. Obstet.* 21:7–10.

2. Van Gelderen, C. J., M. J. England, G. A. Naylor, and T. C. Katzeff. 1986. "Labor in Patients with a Cesarean Section Scar. *S. African. Med. J.* 70:529–532.

3. De Jong, P. 1987. "Trial of Labor Following Cesarean Section—A Study of 212 Patients." *Int. J. Gynecol. Obstet.* 25:405–411.

4. Lahousen, M., and R. Burmucic. 1986. "Zur Frage der Geburtsleitung nach vorausgegangenem Kaiserschnitt." *Geburtsh. u. Frauenheilk.* 46:170–173.

5. Demianczuk, N. N., D. J. S. Hunter, and D. W. Taylor. 1982. "Trial of Labor After Previous Cesarean Section: Prognostic Indicators of Outcome." *Am. J. Obstet. Gynecol.* 142:640–642.

6. Kolle-Frick, M., W. Prinz, and W. D. Jonatha. 1984.

"The Course of Labor Following Cesarean Section." *Geburtsh. u. Frauenheilk.* 44:146–149.

7. Dadak, C., and E. Lasnik. 1985. "The Course of Pregnancy and Fetal Outcome After Cesarean Section. *"Wien. Klin. Wochenschr.* 97(23):880–883.

8. Lawrence, R. 1953. "Vaginal Delivery After Cesarean Section." *J. Obstet. Gynecol. Br. Emp.* 60:237–243.

9. Baker, K. 1955. "Vaginal Delivery After Lower Uterine Cesarean Section." *Surg. Gynecol. Obstet.* 100:690–696.

10. McGarry, J. A. 1969. "The Management of Patients Previously Delivered by Cesarean Section." *Obstet. Gynecol. Brit. Cwlth.* 76:137–143.

11. Meehan, F. P., A. S. Moolgaoker, and J. Stallworthy. 1972. "Vaginal Delivery Under Caudal Analgesia After Cesarean Section." *Brit. Med. J.* 2:740–742.

12. MacKenzie, I. Z., S. Bradley, and M. P. Embrey. 1984. "Vaginal Prostaglandins and Labor Induction for Patients Previously Delivered by Cesarean Section." *Brit. J. Obstet. Gynecol.* 91:7–10.

13. Lao, T. T., and B. F. H. Leung. 1987. "Labor Induction for Planned Vaginal Delivery in Patients with Previous Cesarean Section." *Acta. Obstet. Gynecol. Scand.* 66: 413–416.

14. Dhall, K., S. C. Mittal, V. Grover, and G. I. Dhall. 1987. "Childbirth Following Primary Cesarean Section. *Int. J. Gynecol. Obstet.* 25:199–205.

15. Jain, M., S. Pandey, L. K. Pandey, and D. Sharma. 1987. "Obstetric Prospects After Cesarean Section." *J. Indian. Med. Assoc.* 85(11):324–326.

16. Chi, I. C., A. B. Saifuddin, D. E. Gunatilake, and S. L. Wallace. 1983. "Deliveries After Cesarean Birth in Two Asian Hospitals." *Int. J. Gynecol. Obstet.* 21:11–16.

17. Allahbadia, N. K. 1963. "Vaginal Delivery Following Cesarean Section." *Am. J. Obstet. Gynecol.* 85(2):241–249.

18. Browne, A., and J. McGrath. 1965. "Vaginal Delivery After Previous Cesarean Section: A Survey of 800 Cases at the Rotunda Hospital, Dublin." *Obstet. Gynecol. Br. Emp.* 72:557–565.

19. MacDonald, D. 1982. "Previous Obstetrical or Gynecological Surgery." *Clin. Obstet. Gynecol.* 9(1):147–169.

20. Molloy, B. G., O. Sheil, and M. N. Duignan. 1987. "Delivery After Cesarean Section: Review of 2,176 Consecutive Cases." *Brit. Med. J.* 294:1645–1647.

21. Rudick, V., D. Niv, M. Hetman-Peri, E. Geller, A. Avni, and A. Golan. 1984. "Epidural Analgesia for Planned Vaginal Delivery Following Previous Cesarean Section." *Obstet. Gynecol.* 64:621–623.

22. Weissman, A., P. Jokobi, and E. Zimmer. 1987. "Trial of Labor Without Oxytocin in Patients with Previous Cesarean Section." *Am. J. Perinatology.* 4(2):140–143.

23. Molina, P., A. L. Regalia, A. Scian, P. Spreafico, and E. Colombo. 1985. "Esiti Materni e Neonatali del Parto Vaginale nelle Pazienti con T.C. Pregresso." *Ann. Ost. Gin. Med. Perin.* CVI:165–169.

24. Chattopadhyay, K., B. S. Sengupta, Y. B. Edress, and A. Lambourne. 1988. "Vaginal Birth After Cesarean Section: Management Debate." *Int. J. Gynecol. Obstet.* 26:189–196.

25. Gutierrez, E. B., X. L. Del Campo, and E. P. Wiff. 1984. "Parto Vaginal en Pacientes Portadoras de Histerorrafia." *Rev. Chil. Obstet. Ginecol.* XLIX:434–438.

26. Schneider, J., D. Gallego, and R. Benito. 1988. "Trial of Labor After Earlier Cesarean Section." *J. Reprod. Med.* 33(5):453–456.

27. Carlsson, C., G. Nybell-Lindahl, and I. Ingemarsson. 1980. "Extradural Block in Patients Who Have Previously Undergone Cesarean Section." *Br. J. Anaesth.* 52:827–829.

28. Nielsen, T. F., U. Ljungblad, and H. Hagberg. 1989. "Rupture and Dehiscence of Cesarean Section Scar During Pregnancy and Delivery." *Am. J. Obstet. Gynecol.* 160:569–573.

29. Morewood, G. A., M. J. O'Sullivan, and J. McConney. 1973. "Vaginal Delivery After Cesarean Section." *Obstet. Gynecol.* 42(4):589–595.

30. Delmis, J., and D. Bojanic. 1986. Delivery After Previous Cesarean Section." *Jogosl. Ginekol. Perinatol.* 26: 73–77.

INDEX

About the Author

Dr. Bruce L. Flamm completed undergraduate studies in biochemistry at the University of California at Riverside followed by graduate studies in pharmacology at UCLA. He attended medical school at Wake Forest University in North Carolina and then returned to the University of California where he completed his internship and residency in obstetrics and gynecology. For the past eight years his main interest has been the rapidly rising U.S. cesarean section rate. Dr. Flamm, an assistant clinical professor of obstetrics and gynecology at the University of California, has published several medical reports on cesarean-related topics including the world's largest study of normal birth after cesarean section. Reprints of these reports have been requested by doctors and childbirth educators all over the world.

Dr. Flamm is now the director of a major ten-hospital collaborative study on birth after cesarean section and has recently been interviewed by several newspapers including the *Los Angeles Times* and by several television programs including NBC's "Today Show." He is a diplomate of the American Board of Obstetrics and Gynecology and a fellow of the American College of Obstetricians and Gynecologists. Dr. Flamm and his wife, Janice, a certified nurse–midwife, have attended the births of more than five thousand babies.